IMMUNIZATION SAFETY REVIEW

INFLUENZA VACCINES AND NEUROLOGICAL COMPLICATIONS

Immunization Safety Review Committee
Board on Health Promotion and Disease Prevention

Kathleen Stratton, Donna A. Alamario, Theresa Wizemann,
and Marie C. McCormick, Editors

INSTITUTE OF MEDICINE
OF THE NATIONAL ACADEMIES

THE NATIONAL ACADEMIES PRESS
Washington, D.C.
www.nap.edu

THE NATIONAL ACADEMIES PRESS   500 Fifth Street, N.W.   Washington, DC 20001

NOTICE: The project that is the subject of this report was approved by the Governing Board of the National Research Council, whose members are drawn from the councils of the National Academy of Sciences, the National Academy of Engineering, and the Institute of Medicine. The members of the committee responsible for the report were chosen for their special competences and with regard for appropriate balance.

Support for this project was provided by the Centers for Disease Control and Prevention and the National Institute of Allergy and Infectious Diseases of the National Institutes of Health as part of a National Institutes of Health Task Order No. 74. The views presented in this report are those of the Institute of Medicine Immunization Safety Review Committee and are not necessarily those of the funding agencies.

International Standard Book Number 0-309-09086-5 (Book)
International Standard Book Number 0-309-52781-3 (PDF)

Additional copies of this report are available from the National Academies Press, 500 Fifth Street, N.W., Lockbox 285, Washington, DC 20055; (800) 624-6242 or (202) 334-3313 (in the Washington metropolitan area); Internet, http://www.nap.edu.

For more information about the Institute of Medicine, visit the IOM home page at: **www.iom.edu.**

The serpent has been a symbol of long life, healing, and knowledge among almost all cultures and religions since the beginning of recorded history. The serpent adopted as a logotype by the Institute of Medicine is a relief carving from ancient Greece, now held by the Staatliche Museen in Berlin.

"Knowing is not enough; we must apply.
Willing is not enough; we must do."
—Goethe

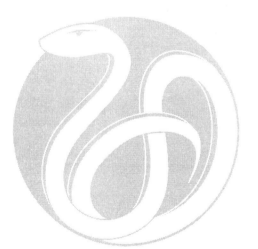

INSTITUTE OF MEDICINE
OF THE NATIONAL ACADEMIES

Shaping the Future for Health

THE NATIONAL ACADEMIES
Advisers to the Nation on Science, Engineering, and Medicine

The **National Academy of Sciences** is a private, nonprofit, self-perpetuating society of distinguished scholars engaged in scientific and engineering research, dedicated to the furtherance of science and technology and to their use for the general welfare. Upon the authority of the charter granted to it by the Congress in 1863, the Academy has a mandate that requires it to advise the federal government on scientific and technical matters. Dr. Bruce M. Alberts is president of the National Academy of Sciences.

The **National Academy of Engineering** was established in 1964, under the charter of the National Academy of Sciences, as a parallel organization of outstanding engineers. It is autonomous in its administration and in the selection of its members, sharing with the National Academy of Sciences the responsibility for advising the federal government. The National Academy of Engineering also sponsors engineering programs aimed at meeting national needs, encourages education and research, and recognizes the superior achievements of engineers. Dr. Wm. A. Wulf is president of the National Academy of Engineering.

The **Institute of Medicine** was established in 1970 by the National Academy of Sciences to secure the services of eminent members of appropriate professions in the examination of policy matters pertaining to the health of the public. The Institute acts under the responsibility given to the National Academy of Sciences by its congressional charter to be an adviser to the federal government and, upon its own initiative, to identify issues of medical care, research, and education. Dr. Harvey V. Fineberg is president of the Institute of Medicine.

The **National Research Council** was organized by the National Academy of Sciences in 1916 to associate the broad community of science and technology with the Academy's purposes of furthering knowledge and advising the federal government. Functioning in accordance with general policies determined by the Academy, the Council has become the principal operating agency of both the National Academy of Sciences and the National Academy of Engineering in providing services to the government, the public, and the scientific and engineering communities. The Council is administered jointly by both Academies and the Institute of Medicine. Dr. Bruce M. Alberts and Dr. Wm. A. Wulf are chair and vice chair, respectively, of the National Research Council.

www.national-academies.org

IMMUNIZATION SAFETY REVIEW COMMITTEE

Reviewers

This report has been reviewed in draft form by individuals chosen for their diverse perspectives and technical expertise, in accordance with procedures approved by the NRC's Report Review Committee. The purpose of this independent review is to provide candid and critical comments that will assist the institution in making its published report as sound as possible and to ensure that the report meets institutional standards for objectivity, evidence, and responsiveness to the study charge. The review comments and draft manuscript remain confidential to protect the integrity of the deliberative process. We wish to thank the following individuals for their review of this report:

Ann Bostrom, Ph.D., Georgia Institute of Technology
Linda D. Cowan, Ph.D., University of Oklahoma
Paul Glezen, M.D., Baylor College of Medicine
Richard T. Johnson, M.D., Johns Hopkins University School of Medicine
Samuel L. Katz, M.D., Duke University Medical Center
Peter H. Meyers, J.D., George Washington University
William Schaffner, M.D., Vanderbilt University School of Medicine
Brian Ward, M.D., McGill University

Although the reviewers listed above have provided many constructive comments and suggestions, they were not asked to endorse the conclusions or recommendations nor did they see the final draft of the report before its release. The review of this report was overseen by **Floyd Bloom, M.D.,** The Scripps Research Institute. Appointed by the National Research Council and Institute of Medicine, he was responsible for making certain that an independent examination of this report was carried out in accordance with institutional procedures and that all review comments were carefully considered. Responsibility for the final content of this report rests entirely with the authoring committee and the institution.

Foreword

Vaccines are among the greatest public health accomplishments of the past century. In recent years, however, a number of concerns have been raised about both the safety of and the need for certain immunizations. Indeed, immunization safety is a contentious area of public health policy, with discourse around it having become increasingly polarized and exceedingly difficult. The numerous controversies and allegations surrounding immunization safety signify an erosion of public trust in those responsible for vaccine research, development, licensure, schedules, and policy making. Because vaccines are so widely used—and because state laws require that children be vaccinated to enter daycare and school, in part to protect others—immunization safety concerns should be vigorously pursued in order to restore this trust.

It is in this context that the Institute of Medicine (IOM) was approached more than a year ago by the Centers for Disease Control and Prevention and the National Institutes of Health to convene an independent committee that could provide timely and objective assistance to the Department of Health and Human Services in reviewing emerging immunization safety concerns.

The IOM was chartered by the National Academy of Sciences in 1970 to serve as an adviser to the federal government on issues affecting the public's health, as well as to act independently in identifying important issues of medical care, research, and education. The IOM thus brings to this mission three decades of experience in conducting independent analyses of significant public health policy issues. In particular, as described in more detail in this report, the IOM has a long history of involvement in vaccine safety. The IOM published its first major vaccine safety report in 1977, followed by a subsequent report in 1988; both focused on the safety of polio vaccines. Two subsequent major reports, published in 1991 and 1994, examined the adverse events of childhood vaccines. Since then, the IOM has conducted several smaller studies and workshops focused on various vaccine safety topics. These studies were all well received by both the public and policy makers, and previous IOM committees on vaccine safety issues have been viewed as objective and credible.

Given the sensitive nature of the present immunization safety review study, the IOM felt it was especially critical to establish strict criteria for committee membership. These criteria prevented participation by anyone with financial ties to vaccine manufacturers or their parent companies, previous service on major vaccine advisory committees, or prior expert testimony or publications on issues of vaccine safety.

The rationale for imposing these stringent criteria was twofold. First, given growing public concern about vaccine safety and the public scrutiny surrounding this committee's work, it was important to establish standards that would preclude any real or perceived conflict of interest or bias on the part of the committee members. While the committee members all share a belief in the benefits of vaccines to the public health, none of them has any vested interest in any of the vaccine safety issues that will come before them. Second, the IOM wanted to ensure consistency in the committee membership and to avoid having members recuse themselves from the deliberations because they had participated in the development or evaluation of a vaccine under study.

Thus, the IOM has convened a distinguished panel of 15 members who possess significant breadth and depth of expertise in a number of fields, including pediatrics, neurology, immunology, internal medicine, infectious diseases, genetics, epidemiology, biostatistics, risk perception and communication, decision analysis, public health, nursing, and ethics. The committee members were chosen because they are leading authorities in their respective fields, are well respected by their colleagues, and have no conflicts of interest. This committee brought a fresh perspective to these critically important issues and approached its charge with impartiality and scientific rigor.

The IOM does not propose the use of the criteria it has laid out above in selecting members for federal vaccine advisory committees. The IOM committee was convened for a very different purpose from the usual federal vaccine advisory committees and, as such, required different standards.

As with all reports from the IOM, the committee's work was reviewed by an independent panel of experts. The purpose of the review process is to enhance the clarity, cogency, and accuracy of the final report and to ensure that the authors and the IOM are creditably represented by the report published in their names. The report review process is overseen by the National Research Council's (NRC) Report Review Committee (RRC), comprised of approximately 30 members of the National Academy of Sciences, National Academy of Engineering, and IOM. The IOM, in conjunction with the RRC, appoints a panel of reviewers with a diverse set of perspectives on key issues considered in the report. Unlike the selection criteria for committee membership (discussed above), many reviewers will have strong opinions and biases about the report topic. The composition of the review panel is not disclosed to the committee until after the report is approved for release. While the committee must consider and evaluate all comments from reviewers, it is not obligated to change its report in response to the reviewers' comments. The committee must, however, justify its responses to the reviewers' comments to the satisfaction of the RRC's review monitor and the IOM's review coordinator. A report may not be released to the sponsors or the public, nor may its findings be disclosed, until after the review process has been satisfactorily completed and all authors have approved the revised draft.

This report represents the unanimous conclusions and recommendations of that dedicated committee whose members deliberated a critical health issue. The report's conclusions and recommendations should be of value to all concerned about these important matters.

Harvey V. Fineberg
President, Institute of Medicine

Acknowledgments

The committee would like to acknowledge the many speakers and attendees at its open meeting held on March 13, 2003, at the Hotel Monaco in Washington, D.C. The discussions were informative and helpful. The committee would also like to thank those people who submitted information to the committee through the mail or via e-mail. Finally, the committee would like to thank the IOM staff for their dedication to this project. Without their commitment, attention to detail, creativity, sensitivity, and hard work, this project would be unworkable.

Contents

Executive Summary

ABSTRACT

Infection with the influenza virus can have a serious effect on the health of people of all ages, although it is particularly worrisome for infants, the elderly, and people with underlying heart or lung problems. At least 35,000 people die in the United States every year from influenza infection. A vaccine exists (the "flu" shot) that can greatly decrease the impact of influenza. Because the strains of virus that are expected to cause serious illness and death are slightly different every year, the vaccine is also slightly different every year and it must be given every year, unlike other vaccines. The influenza vaccine that was used in 1976 for the expected "Swine Flu" epidemic (which never materialized) was associated with cases of a nervous system condition called Guillain-Barré syndrome (GBS). Ever since that time, public health leaders, doctors and nurses, and the public have wondered whether every year's influenza vaccine can cause GBS or other similar conditions.

The Immunization Safety Review committee reviewed the data on influenza vaccine and neurological conditions and concluded that the evidence favored acceptance of a causal relationship between the 1976 swine influenza vaccine and GBS in adults. The evidence about GBS for other years' influenza vaccines is not clear one way or the other (that is, the evidence is inadequate to accept or reject a causal relationship).

The committee concluded that the evidence favored rejection of a causal relationship between influenza vaccines and exacerbation of multiple sclerosis. For the other neurological conditions studied, the committee concluded the evidence about the effects of influenza vaccine is inadequate to accept or reject a causal relationship. The committee also reviewed theories on how the influ-

1

enza vaccine could damage the nervous system. The evidence was at most weak that the vaccine could act in humans in ways that could lead to these neurological problems. See Box ES-1 for a summary of all recommendations and conclusions.

Immunization to protect children and adults from many infectious diseases is one of the greatest achievements of public health. Immunization is not without risks, however. Given the widespread use of vaccines, state mandates requiring vaccination of children for entry into day care, school, or college, and the importance of ensuring that trust in immunization programs is justified, it is essential that safety concerns receive assiduous attention.

The Immunization Safety Review Committee was established by the Institute of Medicine (IOM) to evaluate the evidence on possible causal associations between immunizations and certain adverse outcomes, and to then present conclusions and recommendations. The committee's mandate also includes assessing the broader societal significance of these immunization safety issues. While the committee members all share the view that immunization is generally beneficial, none of them has a vested interest in the specific immunization safety issues that come before the group.

The committee reviews three immunization safety review topics each year, addressing one at a time. In this seventh report in the series, the committee examines the hypothesis that influenza vaccines are associated with an increased risk of neurological complications, particularly Guillain-Barré syndrome (GBS) and multiple sclerosis (MS).

The committee is charged with assessing both the scientific evidence regarding the hypotheses under review and the significance of the issues for society:

• The *scientific* assessment has two components: an examination of the epidemiologic and clinical evidence regarding a possible *causal relationship* between exposure to the vaccine and the adverse event; and an examination of theory and experimental evidence from human or animal studies regarding biological *mechanisms* that might be relevant to the hypothesis.

• The *significance* assessment addresses such considerations as the burden of the health risks associated with the vaccine-preventable disease and with the adverse event. Other considerations may include the perceived intensity of public or professional concern, or the feasibility of additional research to help resolve scientific uncertainty regarding causality.

The findings of the scientific and significance assessments provide the basis for the committee's recommendations regarding the public health response to the issues. In particular, the committee addresses needs for a review of immunization policy, for current and future research, and for effective communication strategies.

For its evaluation of the question concerning influenza vaccines and neurological complications, the committee held an open scientific meeting in March

2003 (see Appendix B) to hear presentations on issues germane to the topic. These presentations are available in electronic form (audio files and slides) on the project website (www.iom.edu/imsafety). In addition, the committee reviewed an extensive collection of material, primarily from the published, peer-reviewed scientific and medical literature. A list of the materials reviewed by the committee, including many items not cited in this report, can be found on the project's website.

THE FRAMEWORK FOR SCIENTIFIC ASSESSMENT

Causality

The Immunization Safety Review Committee has adopted the framework for assessing causality developed by previous IOM committees (IOM, 1991; 1994a,b), convened under the congressional mandate of P.L. 99-660 to address questions of immunization safety. The categories of causal conclusions used by the committee are as follows:

1. No evidence
2. Evidence is inadequate to accept or reject a causal relationship
3. Evidence favors rejection of a causal relationship
4. Evidence favors acceptance of a causal relationship
5. Evidence establishes a causal relationship.

Assessments begin from a position of neutrality regarding the specific vaccine safety hypothesis under review. That is, there is no presumption that a specific vaccine (or vaccine component) does or does not cause the adverse event in question. The committee does not conclude that the vaccine does not cause the adverse event merely if the evidence is inadequate to support causality. Instead, it concludes that the "evidence is inadequate to accept or reject a causal relationship."

Biological Mechanisms

Evidence considered in the scientific assessment of biological mechanisms[1] includes human, animal, and *in vitro* studies related to biological or pathophysiological processes by which immunizations could cause an adverse event. When other evidence of causality is available, biological data add supportive evidence but they cannot prove causality on their own.

---

[1]For a discussion of the evolution of the terminology concerning biological mechanisms, see the committee's earlier reports (IOM, 2001a,b; 2002a,b).

4 IMMUNIZATION SAFETY REVIEW

The committee has established three general categories of evidence on biological mechanisms:

1. *Theoretical.* A reasonable mechanism can be hypothesized that is commensurate with scientific knowledge and does not contradict known physical and biological principles, but it has not been demonstrated in whole or in part in humans or in animal models.
2. *Experimental.* A mechanism can be shown to operate in *in vitro* systems, animals, or humans. But, experimental evidence often describes mechanisms that represent only a portion of the pathological process required for expression of disease. Showing that multiple portions of a process operate in reasonable experimental models strengthens the case that the mechanisms could possibly result in disease in humans.
3. *Evidence that the mechanism results in known disease in humans.* For example, the wild-type infection causes the adverse health outcome, or another vaccine has been demonstrated to cause the same adverse outcome by the same or a similar mechanism.

If the committee identifies evidence of biological mechanisms that could be operational, it will offer a summary judgment of that body of evidence as weak, moderate, or strong. The summary judgment of the strength of the evidence also depends both on the quantity (e.g., number of studies or number of subjects in a study) and quality (e.g., the nature of the experimental system or study design) of the evidence.

Influenza Vaccines and Neurological Complications

The committee's review of the evidence concerning risks that might be associated with influenza vaccines had to take into account a distinctive feature of the vaccine: its formulation changes from year to year to reflect changes in the strains of influenza virus circulating in the population. As a result, the question before the committee actually concerns many different influenza vaccines rather than a single, consistent product used over many years. In terms of the neurological outcomes of concern, GBS is the most widely cited. Other outcomes considered by the committee are multiple sclerosis (MS) and optic neuritis.

Influenza and Influenza Vaccines

Influenza is an acute and highly contagious viral respiratory disease that occurs worldwide. Although some infections are subclinical, influenza is responsible for substantial morbidity and mortality. The elderly, young children, and persons with chronic cardiac or pulmonary diseases are generally at greatest risk for fatal complications (Dolin, 2001). In the United States alone, the disease is now estimated to contribute to an average of 36,000 deaths each year, a toll that has risen as the population has aged (Thompson et al., 2003). The extent and severity of influenza infections can vary widely from year to year.

The influenza viruses infects the respiratory epithelium. Onset of illness is often abrupt, with systemic symptoms that include fever, chills, headache, myalgias and respiratory signs such as cough and sore throat. In uncomplicated cases, acute illness typically resolves over 2 to 5 days. Recovery may be complete within a week, but some patients experience persistent weakness or lassitude (Dolin, 2001). Many of the influenza-related deaths result from complications, the most common being secondary bacterial pneumonia. Influenza can also exacerbate chronic pulmonary conditions or contribute to a general deterioration in cardiac or pulmonary function, especially in the elderly or persons with chronic illness.

Influenza viruses are members of the family Orthomyxoviridae. Three forms of the virus—referred to as types A, B, and C—are known to infect humans. The B and C viruses circulate only in humans, with type C producing little illness. Type A viruses, however, circulate not exclusively in humans but also in wild aquatic birds, their natural reservoir. In addition, the type A viruses infect other birds and several species of mammals. Influenza A viruses are subtyped based on antigenic characteristics of their spike-like surface glycoproteins hemagglutinin (HA) and neuraminidase (NA) (Dolin, 2001). Influenza B and C viruses also carry HA and NA surface antigens, but they are not given subtype designations.

Immunity to influenza depends on the formation of antibodies to the glyco-protein surface antigens HA and NA (Dolin, 2001; Hilleman, 2002). However, influenza viruses of types A and B are successful in evading pre-existing immunity from prior infections or vaccination because HA and NA continuously evolve (Dolin, 2001; CDC, 2002a). Replication of the genetic material in the influenza A and B virus genomes is error-prone and there is no proofreading mechanism, allowing for the accumulation of point mutations (Dolin, 2001; Hilleman, 2002; Steinhauer and Skehel, 2002; Ziegler and Cox, 1999). Such mutations in the genes encoding the surface antigens lead to what is called antigenic drift. The influenza A virus is also subject to antigenic shift—a major change in the HA or NA antigens (e.g., from H1 to H2 or N1 to N2). Antigenic drift occurs often, leading the need for annual influenza vaccination. Antigenic shift occurs less frequently and is associated with increases in morbidity and mortality.

Vaccination is the primary means of reducing the impact of influenza. The effectiveness of influenza vaccines depends, in part, on the match between the viral strains used to produce them and the strains that actually circulate in the subsequent influenza season. The Advisory Committee on Immunization Practices (ACIP) currently recommends influenza vaccination for persons 6 months of age and older who are at increased risk for complications of influenza, all persons 50 to 64 years old, and health care workers and others who can routinely transmit influenza to those at high risk for complications (CDC, 2003c). Persons considered to be at high risk for complications from influenza include persons aged 65 years or older; residents of nursing homes and chronic care facilities; children and adults with chronic lung, heart, kidney, metabolic, or immune system disorders; and women who will be in the second or third trimester of pregnancy during influenza season. The ACIP encourages, when feasible, the use of influenza vaccine for children 6 to 23 months of age.

The majority of influenza vaccines currently approved for use in the United States are inactivated ("killed virus").[2] A live attenuated intranasal influenza vaccine was just approved by the FDA in June 2003 for use in the United States in healthy individuals aged 5-49 years (DHHS, 2003). Current vaccines are trivalent, produced using strains of influenza A(H1N1), influenza A(H3N2), and influenza B viruses. Because of the continuing antigenic changes in these viruses, new influenza vaccines are formulated each year based on information on the viral strains that circulated during the previous season or are circulating at the time in other parts of the world.

Adverse Neurological Events

The adverse events considered in this report—GBS, MS, and optic neuritis— are primarily diseases involving demyelination of nerve cell axons in either the central (CNS) or peripheral (PNS) nervous systems.

GBS is an acute, immune-mediated paralytic disorder of the peripheral nervous system. Estimates of the annual incidence of GBS range from 0.4 to 4.0 cases per 100,000 population, with most studies pointing to a level of from 1 to 2 cases per 100,000 (Hughes and Rees, 1997; Magira et al., 2003). GBS occurs throughout the year, and in the United States the condition is more likely to occur in adults than in children (Asbury, 2000).

About two-thirds of GBS cases occur several days or weeks after an infectious event (Hughes and Rees, 1997), commonly a diarrheal illness or a virus-like upper-respiratory infection. From 20 percent to 40 percent of all GBS cases are associated with *Campylobacter jejuni* infections (Buzby et al., 1997). Exposure to certain vaccines has also been associated with an increased risk for GBS. The potential association between GBS and influenza vaccines, most notably the 1976 swine influenza vaccine, has been widely studied and is the subject of this report.

The characteristic clinical feature of GBS is an acute, rapidly progressive, symmetrical weakness, with loss of deep tendon reflexes, possible tingling in the feet and hands, and muscle aches (myalgia). Approximately 85 percent of patients will return to normal functioning within 6 to 9 months, but some patients experi-

---

[2]Inactivated influenza vaccines licensed for use in the United States for the 2002 influenza season included FluShield (Wyeth Lederle); Fluvirin (Evans Vaccines, Ltd.); and Fluzone (Aventis Pasteur). As of November 2002, Wyeth ceased producing FlueShield. The live attenuated vaccine FluMist is manufactured by MedImmune Vaccines, Inc and marketed by Wyeth Vaccines.

ence relapses or a prolonged disease course with residual neurological deficits (Asbury, 2000; Joseph and Tsao, 2002). The mortality rate is 3-5 percent, with patients succumbing to undetected respiratory failure, malfunction of the autonomic nervous system, or to complications of immobility such as sepsis or pulmonary embolism (Joseph and Tsao, 2002).

MS affects between 250,000 and 350,000 people in the United States and is the most common inflammatory demyelinating disease of the CNS (Keegan and Noseworthy, 2002). Its incidence and manifestations vary within the population. The relapsing-remitting form, for example, occurs predominantly in females (~1.6:1), but follows a more severe clinical course in males (Noseworthy et al., 2000). The incidence of the disease is highest in persons between the ages of 20 and 40 years, but it is also diagnosed in children as young as 2 years and in older individuals. The prevalence of the disease is between 50 and 250 cases per 100,000 population in high-risk areas such as the Scandinavian countries or the northern United States, whereas it is less than 5 cases per 100,000 in Africa and Japan (Waubant and Stuve, 2002).

Clinically, MS is characterized by a variety of neurological signs and symptoms, reflecting the occurrence of inflammatory demyelinating lesions throughout the CNS. Common presenting symptoms include focal sensory deficits, focal weakness, a loss of vision, double vision, imbalance, and fatigue. The severity of the disease can range from subclinical forms that are diagnosed only after death from other causes to hyperacute forms that lead to death within the first few months after disease onset. The cause of MS remains elusive, but disease susceptibility appears to involve both genetic and environmental factors. Genetic factors are reflected in an increased risk of developing MS among family members of MS patients.

Optic neuritis is caused by an inflammation of the optic nerve, with lesions occurring behind the orbit but anterior to the optic chiasm (IOM, 1994a). Symptoms include rapid vision loss, pain associated with eye movement, dimmed vision, abnormal color vision, altered depth perception, and Uhthoff's phenomenon (visual loss associated with an increase in body temperature) (IOM, 2001c). The majority of cases resolve within a few weeks to months of onset. Optic neuritis can occur as an isolated monophasic disease, or it may be a symptom of other demyelinating diseases such as acute disseminated encephalomyelitis (ADEM) or MS.

SCIENTIFIC ASSESSMENT

Causality

Guillain-Barré Syndrome

For its review of the epidemiologic evidence regarding a possible association between influenza vaccination and GBS, the committee separated studies concerning the vaccines administered during the 1976 National Influenza Immunization Program from studies concerning influenza vaccines administered in subsequent years. The committee reviewed studies that presented data for the nation as a whole and studies based on data for individual states or for military personnel. Case reports were also reviewed, but the committee concluded that reports to VAERS and other case reports submitted to the committee are uninformative with respect to causality, although they are useful for hypothesis generation. Case reports help describe the domain of concerns, but the data are usually uncorroborated clinical descriptions that are insufficient to permit meaningful comment or to contribute to a causality argument. The analytical value of data from VAERS and other passive surveillance systems is limited by such problems as underreporting, lack of detail, inconsistent diagnostic criteria, and inadequate denominator data (Ellenberg and Chen, 1997; Singleton et al., 1999).

1976 Swine Influenza Vaccine

Studies that examined the association between swine influenza vaccine and GBS, including analysis and reanalysis of nationwide data (Schonberger et al 1979, Langmuir et al 1984), and state-based studies (Parkin et al., 1978; Marks and Halpin, 1980; Breman and Hayner, 1984; Safranek et al., 1991) consistently showed an increased risk of GBS for the vaccinated population (See Table 3). **The committee concludes that the evidence favors acceptance of a causal relationship between 1976 swine influenza vaccine and Guillain-Barré syndrome in adults.** Concerns that the evidence of increased risk found in the original analysis of the national data might have been a reflection of inaccuracies in ascertainment of GBS cases have been addressed in subsequent studies by detailed and systematic reviews of clinical data to verify GBS diagnoses.

Although the studies of GBS among military personnel (Johnson, 1982; Kurland et al., 1986) do not show an association with the 1976 swine influenza vaccine, these studies have limitations that led the committee to discount their findings in its evaluation of the evidence. Military personnel represent a more limited age range than the civilian population and are typically healthier on average than civilians of comparable ages. In addition, information bias may have been present because estimates of the number of vaccinations administered and the number of people serving in the military were not validated and the accuracy of the data sources was not reported. Thus, these studies are limited in their ability to contribute to the causality argument.

Influenza Vaccines Used after 1976

The committee reviewed several population-based surveillance studies (Hurwitz et al., 1981; Kaplan et al., 1982, Lasky et al., 1998), a study of military personnel (Roscelli et al., 1991), and two unpublished studies that were discussed by Chen (2003) at the committee's public meeting (see Table 4). Their findings were mixed. The studies differed in terms of their design, the case definitions for GBS, their methods of case ascertainment, the size of the study populations, and the influenza seasons covered. Compared with the 1976 immunization experience, vaccinations were administered over a longer period of time in the years covered by these studies, making it more difficult to detect any increase that might have occurred in a rare condition like GBS. Although immunization rates were estimated to be much higher among U.S. Army personnel (Roscelli et al., 1991), the relatively small size of the population vaccinated each year would make detection of vaccine-attributable risk difficult. Because of the nature of case reports, the information from VAERS added little to the committee's ability to assess causality.

The committee concludes that the evidence is inadequate to accept or reject a causal relationship between GBS in adults and influenza vaccines administered after 1976 (that is, subsequent to the swine influenza vaccine program).

Multiple Sclerosis

The committee examined reports on epidemiological studies of relapses among MS patients following influenza vaccination; separately it examined a smaller set of reports concerning the risk of MS onset. All these studies concerned influenza vaccines used in various years, including the swine influenza vaccines of 1976. The committee was also provided with VAERS summary information (Haber, 2003). Reports from passive surveillance systems like VAERS are of little assistance in assessing causality.

On the basis of the Confavreaux study (2001) and the consistent findings from the other studies (Miller et al., 1997; Mokhtarian, 1997; Bamford et al., 1978; Myers et al., 1977), **the committee concludes that the evidence favors rejection of a causal relationship between influenza vaccines and relapse of multiple sclerosis in adults.** Uncontrolled studies and case series (De Keyser et al., 1998; Salvetti et al., 1995; Sibley et al., 1976) provide similar findings, but given their nature they are of limited value in assessing causality. The occurrence of relapse is rare and the power to detect increased risk is limited.

Few studies have examined the association between influenza vaccination and the onset of MS. Only one study (DeStefano et al., 2003) provided a thorough description of the study methods and outcomes. It found no increase in the risk of onset of MS associated with influenza vaccination, but in the absence of confirmation from other sources, **the committee concludes that the evidence is inadequate to accept or reject a causal relationship between influenza vaccines and incident MS in adults.** However, the biological mechanisms involved in the onset of MS are presumed to be related to those involved in relapse. With the epidemiological data favoring the rejection of a causal relationship between influenza vaccines and relapse of MS, the committee sees no reason to suspect that a causal relationship might exist between influenza vaccines and onset of MS. Because the available studies did not consistently report ages (some did not report age at all, and detail is lacking in studies that did report age, for example, reporting average age without a range) and none of the studies specifically included children, the committee could not reach a conclusion on causality in the children's age group, but it also could not clearly define the lower age limit for its conclusion in adults.

Optic Neuritis

With a single epidemiologic study available (DeStefano et al., 2003), **the committee concludes that the evidence is inadequate to accept or reject a causal relationship between influenza vaccines and optic neuritis in adults.** VAERS data and case reports have limited value in assessments of causality. Because the available studies that examined optic neuritis did not specifically include children, the committee could not reach a conclusion on causality in the children's age group, but also could not clearly define the lower age limit for its conclusion in adults.

Other Demyelinating Neurological Conditions

Several case reports have been published mentioning the occurrence of other neurological disorders (e.g., acute disseminated encephalomyelitis, transverse myelitis) after influenza vaccination (Saito et al., 1980; Yahr and Lobo-Antunes, 1972; Bakshi and Mazziotta, 1996; Larner and Farmer, 2000). Other neurological conditions were reported from the surveillance system set-up during the 1976 National Influenza Immunization Program, but the data were not sufficient to assess causality (Retailliau et al., 1980). No other epidemiological studies were identified. Based on the nature of case reports and the paucity of epidemiological data, **the committee concludes that the evidence is inadequate to accept or reject a causal relationship between influenza vaccines and other demyelinating neurological disorders.**

Children and Influenza Vaccines

Influenza vaccine is generally administered to adults, and relatively few studies have reported data concerning any neurological complications observed in children. Currently, ACIP encourages influenza immunization for children ages 6-23 months (CDC, 2003c). A recommendation for annual routine influenza immunization in that age group may be made within the near future (CDC, 2003c). Given concerns that demyelinating neurological disorders might follow receipt of influenza vaccines, the committee describes the relevant data in children, specifically focusing on the age group 6-23 months .

The published reports concerning the 1976 swine influenza vaccine and GBS (Schonberger et al., 1979; Marks and Halpin, 1980; Breman and Hayner, 1984) and the reports on the safety of trivalent inactivated influenza vaccine in children (Neuzil et al., 2001; Gonzalez et al., 2000; Piedra et al., 1993) did not directly examine the relationship between influenza vaccines and demyelinating neurological disorders in children. These studies use a broad and varied definition of "children," and the small number of children in the studies limit the ability to detect rare neurological outcomes, such as GBS and MS. The committee reviewed one unpublished study that reported no cases of MS or other demyelinating disorders in children (France, 2003), but the unpublished nature of the study and the small number of cases limit its use in assessing causality. No published studies directly examined receipt of influenza vaccines and the occurrence of demyelinating neurological disorders in children. Thus, based on the lack of direct published evidence on influenza vaccines and demyelinating neurological disorders in children, especially those aged 6-23 months, **the committee concludes that there is no evidence bearing on a causal relationship between influenza vaccines and demyelinating neurological disorders in children aged 6-23 months.**

Biological Mechanisms

In its assessment of the possibility of a relationship between influenza vaccines and neurological complications, the committee hypothesized two general ways vaccine could lead to neurological complications: immune-mediated processes and neurotoxic effects.

Infection can induce immune-mediated tissue injury. In most cases, this injury is short-lived and resolves as the immune system eliminates active infection. The injury is a consequence of the immune response to the foreign invader, and when the invader is eliminated, the damaging immune process ceases. In some diseases, however, infection appears to induce an injurious immune response in the form of T and B cells that are directed, at least in part, against self antigens. This autoimmune injury must be distinguished from immune-mediated injury that results from persistent but undetected infection.

The two major mechanisms proposed to account for the activation of self-reactive T and B cells and the induction of autoimmunity by infection are molecular mimicry and bystander activation (see IOM 2002b for a complete review of this issue). *Molecular mimicry* is a mechanism by which an antigenic epitope from an infectious agent or other exogenous substance that is structurally similar to (mimics) an epitope of a self-molecule has the potential to trigger the activation of self-reactive, naïve T or B lymphocytes. *Bystander activation* results when an infection creates environmental conditions that allow the activation of self-reactive T and B cells that are normally held in check. For example, tissue damage from an infection (or an inflammatory process) can lead to the liberation or exposure of host antigens in a context that allows for presentation to, activation of, and expansion of self-reactive lymphocytes.

It is conceivable that vaccine antigens could mimic self (host), that stimulation from vaccines could trigger bystander activation just as an infectious organism does, and that either or both of these potentially damaging mechanisms could possibly lead to the development of central or peripheral demyelinating disease. There is no reason in theory why influenza virus antigens, or other substances in the vaccines (e.g., residual traces of constituents from the production process), could not function in this way. Thus, there is a theoretical basis for influenza vaccines to induce immune responses that could possibly lead to demyelination. As discussed in the subsequent section, however, the evidence in support of this theory is limited, and some is indirect.

The following biological evidence relates to the theory that influenza vaccines could be associated with neurological complications:

- **Bystander activation.** Animal models (Hjorth et al., 1984; Ziegler et al., 1983) show that under contrived experimental conditions inoculation with influenza vaccines in combination with myelin antigens (as tissue or gangliosides) leads to demyelinating diseases similar in many respects to GBS. Animal models of MS-like CNS demyelination also exist but have not been linked to influenza viruses or vaccines. In models of peripheral demyelination (EAN-like disease and EN), influenza vaccines had adjuvant properties in the presence of neural antigens. For this model to operate during routine human use of influenza vaccine, neural injury would have to be initiated during the immunization process to release neural antigens with which the vaccine would act as adjuvant, or influenza vaccines would have to contain myelin (which has not been shown) or other components that mimic myelin.

- **Molecular mimicry.** Evidence related to molecular mimicry is mixed.

1. No direct evidence shows that influenza antigens or other vaccine components act as molecular mimics of self antigens in the nervous system. Although two older studies demonstrated similarities in amino acid sequences between the myelin protein P2 and the influenza A virus protein NS2, there is no evidence that this sequence similarity leads to structural similarity or that NS2 can elicit host autoantibodies. In addition, NS2 is not likely to be found in influenza vaccines.

2. A strong set of data indicate that *C. jejuni* antigens can trigger GBS through molecular mimicry. Influenza vaccines are made using viruses cultivated in eggs, and eggs can be contaminated with *C. jejuni*. Although the production of the 1976 swine influenza vaccine by four different manufacturers with four different proprietary seed viruses and different egg sources makes widespread *C. jejuni* contamination seem highly

unlikely, the available evidence cannot exclude the possibility that *C. jejuni* antigens were present in the vaccines from all four manufacturers.

The committee concludes that there is weak evidence for biological mechanisms related to immune-mediated processes, including molecular mimicry and bystander activation, by which receipt of any influenza vaccine could possibly influence an individual's risk of developing the neurological complications of GBS, MS, or other demyelinating conditions such as optic neuritis. In the absence of experimental or human evidence regarding the direct neurotoxic effect of influenza vaccines, the committee concludes that this mechanism is only theoretical.

SIGNIFICANCE ASSESSMENT

The committee considered the significance of the concern that influenza vaccines might increase the risk of developing neurological complications such as GBS or MS. The scientific assessment provided support for a link between GBS and the 1976 influenza vaccines, but the evidence for other outcomes or for vaccines for other years was inadequate to support a conclusion or favored no association. Vaccination plays a key role in efforts to reduce the annual impact of influenza infections, making it important that any vaccine-related risks be identified and evaluated.

Influenza vaccine is an essential tool for reducing the substantial burden of morbidity and mortality associated with influenza infections each year. Not only is the yearly disease toll high, but the prospect of an influenza pandemic is a serious concern to many. If the viral strains used to produce the vaccine are closely matched to the viral strains circulating during the influenza season, vaccination may prevent illness (although not necessarily infection) in 70 to 90 percent of healthy children as young as 6 months of age and healthy adults under age 65. (CDC, 2002b). Vaccination is only 30 to 40 percent effective in preventing illness in older and more frail individuals, but it is 50 to 60 percent effective in preventing hospitalization and 80 percent effective in preventing deaths (CDC, 2002a).

Influenza vaccine must be given every year and is recommended for large segments of the population, making it the one of the most widely used vaccines in the United States. Because the vaccine is used so widely and may be recommended for regular administration to young children, the possibility of vaccine-related adverse events must be given serious consideration. In its scientific assessment, the committee found support for a causal association between the vaccine used in 1976 and GBS. But it found no support for an association with relapses of MS, and inconclusive evidence regarding influenza vaccines used in other years and other neurological conditions. The committee found no evidence bearing on a causal relationship between influenza vaccines and demyelinating neurological disorders in children aged 6-23 months. GBS is a serious condition, but it is rare and the additional risk related to vaccination in 1976 translated into fewer than 6 cases per million vaccinees (Langmuir et al., 1984). By contrast, influenza contributes to an annual average of 13.8 deaths per 100,000 (36,000 deaths, majority are 65 years of age or older) and to an annual excess of 49 pneumonia and influenza related hospitalizations per 100,000 (114,000 hospitalizations) (Thompson et al., 2003; Simonsen et al., 2000). It is important to fully understand any risk for GBS or other neurological complication that might be associated with influenza vaccination to ensure that it can be appropriately weighed against the sizable burden of illness associated with influenza infections.

RECOMMENDATIONS FOR PUBLIC HEALTH RESPONSE

Policy Review

The committee does not recommend a policy review of the recommendations for influenza vaccination by any of the national or federal vaccine advisory bodies on the basis of concerns about neurological complications. Current and future immunization policies should continue to reflect the benefits of influenza vaccination.

Research

With a vaccine as widely used as influenza vaccine, the committee considers it important to pursue research and research-related activities aimed at ensuring that any risk of GBS or other neurological complications is minimized.

Surveillance and Epidemiological Studies

Even though use of the vaccine generally appears to pose minimal risk of adverse neurological events, the strong association between the 1976 vaccine and GBS points to the need for appropriate vigilance through adequate surveillance systems and for better tools to support studies of rare adverse events. **The committee recommends increased surveillance of adverse events associated with influenza vaccination of children, with particular attentiveness to detecting and assessing potential neurological complications. Enhanced surveillance should be in place before an ACIP recommendation is implemented for universal annual influenza vaccination of young children.**

Better methods are needed to identify and assess risks for rare outcomes such as the neurological complications considered in this report. The scale of the 1976 vaccination program helped make detection of the link with GBS feasible. **The committee recommends efforts to develop techniques for the detection and evaluation of rare adverse events and encourages the use of administrative** databases and the standardization of immunization records as part of this effort.

Basic and Clinical Science

Despite improvements over the past 25 years in the broad understanding of the pathogenesis of autoimmune diseases, and of GBS in particular, the exact mechanisms by which the 1976 influenza vaccine precipitated this adverse outcome remain unknown. To gain further insight into these mechanisms, the committee sees a need for additional basic and clinical research on influenza viruses, the composition and immunological properties of the 1976 vaccine, immunological responses to vaccines in general, and host characteristics that may affect susceptibility to adverse events.

There is a need to better understand the immunological responses in recipients of the 1976 swine influenza vaccine who experienced GBS. One avenue of inquiry should be the pathogenesis of influenza viruses in general and the swine influenza strain (A/New Jersey/76) in particular to learn whether and how strains might differ in their ability or predisposition to produce neurological injury. **The committee supports ongoing research aimed at better understanding the pathogenesis of influenza and encourages efforts to anticipate which strains might be more neurologically active.**

Although the 1976 influenza vaccine was produced under atypical conditions, with the four manufacturers given less time than usual while being asked to produce much larger quantities than in previous years, there is no evidence that the speed of manufacture or volume of production produced lapses that could have led to a faulty vaccine. The increased risk of GBS associated with the 1976 swine influenza vaccine appeared consistent for vaccine from the four different manufacturers, for the monovalent and bivalent vaccines, and for the whole- and split-virus vaccines. The consistency of the risk across the sources and types of vaccine argues against, but does not rule out, problems related to the manufacturing process. Issues that might be investigated include whether there was something atypical about the nonviral components of the swine influenza vaccines and, if so, identifying it and determining whether it can be controlled.

The use of eggs to produce vaccine-strain influenza virus suggests the possibility that unrecognized antigens might have been present in the 1976 vaccine. *C. jejuni* infection is a recognized risk factor for GBS, possibly acting through molecular mimicry, and *C. jejuni* commonly infects chickens. Although the committee concluded that molecular mimicry is only theoretically possible as an immune mechanism by which influenza vaccines may cause GBS, the evidence that *C. jejuni* antigens can trigger GBS is strong, and the possibility cannot be excluded that *C. jejuni* antigens were present in swine influenza vaccine from all four manufacturers of the 1976 swine influenza vaccine. **Although stocks of the 1976 vaccine are unlikely available, the committee recommends that if** samples of the influenza vaccines used in 1976 are available, they should be analyzed for the presence of *C. jejuni* antigens, NS1 or NS2 proteins, or other possible contaminants. The 1976 vaccines should be compared with current and other historical influenza vaccines.

Studies in animals (Hjorth et al., 1984; Ziegler et al., 1983) have provided at least some basis for considering bystander activation as a potential mechanism by which influenza vaccines could cause GBS or related neurological complications. As it did in a previous report (IOM, 2002a), the committee recommends continued research using animal and *in vitro* models, as well as with humans, on the mechanisms of immune-mediated neurological diseases that might be associated with exposure to vaccines.

Genetic factors are known to be an important source of variability in the responses of the human immune system and in the risks of autoimmune disease. At present, understanding of the complex interactions among genetic variables and environmental exposures, including vaccines and wild-type infectious organisms, remains incomplete. The committee recommends continued research efforts aimed at identifying genetic variability in human immune system responsiveness as a way to gain a better understanding of genetic susceptibility to vaccine-based adverse events.

Communication

A broader framework for influenza vaccine issues is critical for substantial progress in vaccination rates to be achieved. A rigorous, systematic identification of the influences that affect experts' and subpopulations' views and decisions about vaccines is an important step toward developing such a framework (Bostrom, 1997). Despite the studies that have been conducted to date, a comprehensive context has not yet been compiled for the influenza vaccine. The committee recommends that research be supported to conduct investigations that would deepen and expand the knowledge available from existing studies and more effectively organize what is currently known from these and future projects. Comprehensive influence diagrams of expert and at-risk populations' views of the vaccine are needed to provide a broader context and reveal richer insights than are possible from a review of currently available studies.

BOX ES-1 Committee Conclusions and Recommendations

SCIENTIFIC ASSESSMENT
Causality Conclusions

The committee concludes that the evidence favors acceptance of a causal relationship between 1976 swine influenza vaccine and Guillain-Barré syndrome in adults.

The committee concludes that the evidence is inadequate to accept or reject a causal relationship between GBS in adults and influenza vaccines administered after 1976 (that is, subsequent to the swine influenza vaccine program).

The committee concludes that the evidence favors rejection of a causal relationship between influenza vaccines and relapse of multiple sclerosis in adults.

The committee concludes that the evidence is inadequate to accept or reject a causal relationship between influenza vaccines and incident MS in adults.

The committee concludes that the evidence is inadequate to accept or reject a causal relationship between influenza vaccines and optic neuritis in adults.

The committee concludes that the evidence is inadequate to accept or reject a causal relationship between influenza vaccines and other demyelinating neurological disorders.

The committee concludes that there is no evidence bearing on a causal relationship between influenza vaccines and demyelinating neurological disorders in children aged 6-23 months.

Biological Mechanisms Conclusions

The committee concludes that there is weak evidence for biological mechanisms related to immune-mediated processes, including molecular mimicry and bystander activation, by which receipt of any influenza vaccine could possibly influence an individual's risk of developing the neurological complications of GBS, MS, or other demyelinating conditions such as optic neuritis.

In the absence of experimental or human evidence regarding the direct neurotoxic effect of influenza vaccines, the committee concludes that this mechanism is only theoretical.

continued

BOX ES-1 continued

PUBLIC HEALTH RESPONSE RECOMMENDATIONS
Policy Review

The committee does not recommend a policy review of the recommendations for influenza vaccination by any of the national or federal vaccine advisory bodies on the basis of concerns about neurological complications. Current and future immunization policies should continue to reflect the benefits of influenza vaccination.

Research

The committee recommends increased surveillance of adverse events associated with influenza vaccination of children, with particular attentiveness to detecting and assessing potential neurological complications. Enhanced surveillance should be in place before an ACIP recommendation is implemented for universal annual influenza vaccination of young children.

The committee recommends efforts to develop techniques for the detection and evaluation of rare adverse events and encourages the use of administrative databases and the standardization of immunization records as part of this effort.

Basic Science and Clinical Research

The committee supports ongoing research aimed at better understanding the pathogenesis of influenza and encourages efforts to anticipate which strains might be more neurologically active.

Although stocks of the 1976 vaccine are unlikely available, the committee recommends that if samples of the influenza vaccines used in 1976 are available, they should be analyzed for the presence of *C. jejuni* antigens, NS1 or NS2 proteins, or other possible contaminants. The 1976 vaccines should be compared with current and other historical influenza vaccines.

The committee recommends continued research using animal and *in vitro* models, as well as with humans, on the mechanisms of immune-mediated neurological diseases that might be associated with exposure to vaccines.

The committee recommends continued research efforts aimed at identifying genetic variability in human immune system responsiveness as a way to gain a better understanding of genetic susceptibility to vaccine-based adverse events.

Communication

The committee recommends that research be supported to conduct investigations that would deepen and expand the knowledge available from existing studies and more effectively organize what is currently known from these and future projects.

REFERENCES

Asbury AK. 2000. New concepts of Guillain-Barré syndrome. *J Child Neurol* 15(3):183–91.

Bakshi R, Mazziotta JC. 1996. Acute transverse myelitis after influenza vaccination: magnetic resonance imaging findings. *J Neuroimaging* 6(4):248–50.

Bamford CR, Sibley WA, Laguna JF. 1978. Swine influenza vaccination in patients with multiple sclerosis. *Arch Neurol* 35(4):242–3.

Bostrom A. 1997. Vaccine risk communication: Lessons from risk perception, decision making and environmental risk communication research. *Risk.*

Breman JG, Hayner NS. 1984. Guillain-Barré syndrome and its relationship to swine influenza vaccination in Michigan, 1976-1977. *Am J Epidemiol* 119(6):880–9.

Buzby JC, Allos BM, Roberts T. 1997. The economic burden of Campylobacter-associated Guillain-Barré syndrome. *J Infect Dis* 176 Suppl 2:S192–7.

CDC. 2002a. *Epidemiology and Prevention of Vaccine-Preventable Diseases 7th Edition.* Public Health Foundation.

CDC. 2002b. Prevention and Control of Influenza: recommendations of the Advisory Committee on Immunization Practices (ACIP); *MMWR Morb Mortal Wkly Rep* 51(RR03):1–31.

CDC. 2003. Prevention and control of influenza: Recomendations of the Advisory Committee on Immunization Practices (ACIP). *MMWR Morb Mortal Wkly Rep* 52 (RR08):1–36.

Chen R. 2003. Presentation to the Immunization Safety Review Committee. *Studies Of Guillain-Barré Syndrome (GBS) After Influenza Vaccination.* National Immunization Program.

Confavreux C, Suissa S, Saddier P, Bourdes V, Vukusic S, for the Vaccines in Multiple Sclerosis Study Group. 2001. Vaccinations and the risk of relapse in multiple sclerosis. *N Engl J Med* 344(5):319–326.

De Keyser J, Zwanikken C, Boon M. 1998. Effects of influenza vaccination and influenza illness on exacerbations in multiple sclerosis. *J Neurol Sci* 159(1):51–3.

Department of Health and Human Services (DHHS). 2003. Product Approval Information. www.fda.gov/cber/approvltr/inflmed061703L.htm

DeStefano F, Verstraeten T, Jackson LA, Okoro C, Benson P, Black S, Shinefield H, Mullooly P, Likosky W, Chen R. 2003. Vaccinations and risk of central nervous system demyelinating diseases in adults. *Arch Neurology* 60:504–509.

Dolin R. 2001. Influenza. Braunwald E, Fauci AS, Kasper DL, Hauser SL, Longo DL, Jameson JL, Eds. *Harrison's Principles of Internal Medicine.* 15th ed. New York: McGraw-Hill. Pp. 1125–30.

Ellenberg S, Chen R. 1997. The complicated task of monitoring vaccine safety. *Public Health Reports.* 1997;112:10-20.

France E. 2003. Safety of the Trivalent Inactivated Influenza Vaccine (TIV) Among Children: A Population-Based Study. *Presentation to the Immunization Safety Review Committee.* Washington, DC.

Gonzalez M, Pirez MC, Ward E, Dibarboure H, Garcia A, Picolet H. 2000. Safety and immunogenicity of a paediatric presentation of an influenza vaccine. *Arch Dis Child* 83(6):488–91.

Haber P. 2003. Influenza Vaccine and Neurological Adverse Events. VAERS 7/1990–1/2003. *Presentation to Immunization Safety Review Committee.* Washington, DC.

Hilleman MR. 2002. Realities and enigmas of human viral influenza: pathogenesis, epidemiology and control. *Vaccine* 20(25-26):3068-87.

Hjorth RN, Bonde GM, Piner E, Hartzell RW, Rorke LB, Rubin BA. 1984. Experimental neuritis induced by a mixture of neural antigens and influenza vaccines. A possible model for Guillain-Barré syndrome. *J Neuroimmunol* 6(1):1–8.

Hughes RA, Rees JH. 1997. Clinical and epidemiologic features of Guillain-Barré syndrome. *J Infect Dis* 176 Suppl 2:S92–8.

Hurwitz ES, Schonberger LB, Nelson DB, Holman RC. 1981. Guillain-Barré syndrome and the 1978–1979 influenza vaccine. *N Engl J Med* 304(26):1557–61.

IOM (Institute of Medicine). 1991. *Adverse Events Following Pertussis and Rubella Vaccines.* Washington DC: National Academy Press.

IOM (Institute of Medicine).1994a. *Adverse Events Associated with Childhood Vaccines: Evidence Bearing on Causality.* Washington DC: National Academy Press.

IOM (Institute of Medicine). 1994b. *DPT Vaccine and Chronic Nervous System Dysfunction: A New Analysis.* Washington DC: National Academy Press.

IOM (Institute of Medicine). 2001a. *Immunization Safety Review: Measles-Mumps-Rubella Vaccine and Autism.* Washington DC: National Academy Press.

IOM (Institute of Medicine). 2001b. *Immunization Safety Review: Thimerosal-Containing Vaccines and Neurodevelopmental Disorders.* Washington DC: National Academy Press.

IOM (Institute of Medicine). 2001c. *Multiple Sclerosis: Current Status and Strategies for the Future.* Washington DC: National Academy Press.

IOM (Institute of Medicine). 2002a. *Immunization Safety Review: Hepatitis B Vaccine and Demyelinating Neurological Disorders.* Washington DC: National Academy Press.

IOM (Institute of Medicine). 2002b. *Immunization Safety Review: Multiple Immunizations and Immune Dysfunction.* Washington DC: National Academy Press.

Johnson DE. 1982. Guillain-Barré syndrome in the US Army. *Arch Neurol* 39(1):21–4.

Joseph SA, Tsao CY. 2002. Guillain-Barré syndrome. *Adolesc Med* 13(3):487–94.

Kaplan JE, Katona P, Hurwitz ES, Schonberger LB. 1982. Guillain-Barré syndrome in the United States, 1979–1980 and 1980-1981. Lack of an association with influenza vaccination. *JAMA* 248(6):698–700.

Keegan BM, Noseworthy JH. 2002. Multiple sclerosis. *Annu Rev Med* 53:285–302.

Kurland LT, Wiederholt WC, Beghe E, Kirkpatrick JW, Potter HG, Armstrong FP. 1986. Guillain-Barré Syndrome Following (A/New Jersy/76) Influenza (Swine Flu) Vaccine: Epidemic or Artifact? Springer-Verlag Berlin Heidelberg.

Langmuir AD, Bregman DJ, Kurland LT, Nathanson N, Victor M. 1984. An epidemiologic and clinical evaluation of Guillain-Barré syndrome reported in association with the administration of swine influenza vaccines. *Am J Epidemiol* 119(6):841–79.

Larner AJ, Farmer SF. 2000. Myelopathy following influenza vaccination in inflammatory CNS disorder treated with chronic immunosuppression. *Eur J Neurol* 7(6):731–3.

Lasky T, Terracciano GJ, Magder L, Koski CL, Ballesteros M, Nash D, Clark S, Haber P, Stolley PD, Schonberger LB, Chen RT. 1998. The Guillain-Barré syndrome and the 1992–1993 and 1993–1994 influenza vaccines. *N Engl J Med* 339(25):1797–1802.

Magira EE, Papaioakim M, Nachamkin I, Asbury AK, Li CY, Ho TW, Griffin JW, McKhann GM, Monos DS. 2003. Differential distribution of HLA-DQ beta/DR beta epitopes in the two forms of Guillain-Barré syndrome, acute motor axonal neuropathy and acute inflammatory demyelinating polyneuropathy (AIDP): identification of DQ beta epitopes associated with susceptibility to and protection from AIDP. *J Immunol* 170(6):3074–80.

Marks JS, Halpin TJ. 1980. Guillain-Barré syndrome in recipients of A/New Jersey influenza vaccine. *JAMA* 243(24):2490-4.

Miller AE, Morgante LA, Buchwald LY, Nutile SM, Coyle PK, Krupp LB, Doscher CA, Lublin FD, Knobler RL, Trantas F, Kelley L, Smith CR, La Rocca N, Lopez S. 1997. A multicenter, randomized, double-blind, placebo-controlled trial of influenza immunization in multiple sclerosis. *Neurology* 48(2):312–4.

Mokhtarian F, Shirazian D, Morgante L, Miller A, Grob D, Lichstein E. 1997. Influenza virus vaccination of patients with multiple sclerosis. *Mult Scler* 3(4):243–7.

Myers LW, Ellison GW, Lucia M, Novom S, Holevoet M, Madden D, Sever J, Noble GR. 1977. Swine influenza virus vaccination in patients with multiple sclerosis. *J Infect Dis* 136 Suppl:S546–54.

Neuzil KM, Dupont WD, Wright PF, Edwards KM. 2001. Efficacy of inactivated and cold-adapted vaccines against influenza A infection, 1985 to 1990: the pediatric experience. *Pediatr Infect Dis J* 20(8):733–40.

Noseworthy JH, Lucchinetti C, Rodriguez M, Weinshenker BG. 2000. Multiple sclerosis. *N Engl J Med* 343(13):938–52.

Parkin WE, Beecham HJ, Streiff E, Sharrar RG, Harris JC. 1978. Relationship studied in Pennsylvania. Guillain-Barré syndrome and influenza immunization. *Pa Med* 81(4):47–8, 50–2.

Piedra PA, Glezen WP, Mbawuike I, Gruber WC, Baxter BD, Boland FJ, Byrd RW, Fan LL, Lewis JK, Rhodes LJ. 1993. Studies on reactogenicity and immunogenicity of attenuated bivalent cold recombinant influenza type A (CRA) and inactivated trivalent influenza virus (TI) vaccines in infants and young children. *Vaccine* 11(7):718–24.

Retailliau HF, Curtis AC, Storr G, Caesar G, Eddins DL, Hattwick MA. 1980. Illness after influenza vaccination reported through a nationwide surveillance system, 1976–1977. *Am J Epidemiol* 111(3):270–8.

Roscelli JD, Bass JW, Pang L. 1991. Guillain-Barré syndrome and influenza vaccination in the US Army, 1980– 1988. *Am J Epidemiol* 133(9):952–5.

Safranek TJ, Lawrence DN, Kurland LT, Culver DH, Wiederholt WC, Hayner NS, Osterholm MT, O'Brien P, Hughes JM. 1991. Reassessment of the association between Guillain-Barré syndrome and receipt of swine influenza vaccine in 1976–1977: results of a two-state study. Expert Neurology Group. *Am J Epidemiol* 133(9):940–51.

Saito H, Endo M, Takase S, Itahara K. 1980. Acute disseminated encephalomyelitis after influenza vaccination. *Arch Neurol* 37(9):564–6.

Salvetti M, Pisani A, Bastianello S, Millefiorini E, Buttinelli C, Pozzilli C. 1995. Clinical and MRI assessment of disease activity in patients with multiple sclerosis after influenza vaccination. *J Neurol* 242(3):143–6.

Schonberger LB, Bregman DJ, Sullivan-Bolyai JZ, Keenlyside RA, Ziegler DW, Retailliau HF, Eddins DL, Bryan JA. 1979. Guillain-Barré syndrome following vaccination in the National Influenza Immunization Program, United States, 1976–1977. *Am J Epidemiol* 110(2):105–23.

Sibley WA, Bamford CR, Laguna JF. 1976. Influenza vaccination in patients with multiple sclerosis. *JAMA* 236(17):1965–6.

Singleton JA, Lloyd JC, Mootrey GT, Salive ME, Chen RT. 1999. An overview of the vaccine adverse event reporting system (VAERS) as a surveillance system. *Vaccine* 17:2908-2917.

Thompson WW, Shay DK, Weintraub E, Brammer L, Cox N, Anderson LJ, Fukuda K. 2003. Mortality associated with influenza and respiratory syncytial virus in the United States. *JAMA* 289(2):179–86.

Waubant E, Stuve O. 2002. Suspected mechanisms involved in multiple sclerosis and putative role of hepatitis B vaccine in multiple sclerosis. *Commissioned background paper for IOM Immunization Safety Review Committee.*

Yahr MD, Lobo-Antunes J. 1972. Relapsing encephalomyelitis following the use of influenza vaccine. *Arch Neurol* 27(2):182–3.

Ziegler DW, Gardner JJ, Warfield DT, Walls HH. 1983. Experimental allergic neuritis-like disease in rabbits after injection with influenza vaccines mixed with gangliosides and adjuvants. *Infect Immun* 42(2):824–30.

Ziegler T, Cox NJ. 1999. Influenza viruses. In: Murray PR, Baron EJ, Pfaller MA, Tenover FC, Yolken, eds. *Manual of Clinical Microbiology.* 7th ed. Washington, DC: ASM Press.

Immunization Safety Review: Influenza Vaccines and Neurological Complications

Immunization to protect children and adults from many infectious diseases is one of the greatest achievements of public health. Immunization is not without risks, however. It is well established, for example, that the oral polio vaccine on rare occasion has caused paralytic polio and that vaccines sometimes produce anaphylactic shock. Given the widespread use of vaccines, state mandates requiring vaccination of children for entry into school, college, or day care, and the importance of ensuring that trust in immunization programs is justified, it is essential that safety concerns receive assiduous attention.

The Immunization Safety Review Committee was established by the Institute of Medicine (IOM) to evaluate the evidence on possible causal associations between immunizations and certain adverse outcomes, and to then present conclusions and recommendations. The committee's mandate also includes assessing the broader significance for society of these immunization safety issues.

This seventh report from the committee examines the hypothesis that influenza vaccines are associated with an increased risk of neurological complications, particularly Guillain-Barré syndrome (GBS) and multiple sclerosis (MS).

THE CHARGE TO THE COMMITTEE

Challenges to the safety of immunizations are prominent in public and scientific debate. Given these persistent and growing concerns about immunization safety, the Centers for Disease Control and Prevention (CDC) and the National Institutes of Health (NIH) recognized the need for an independent, expert group to address immunization safety in a timely and objective manner. The IOM has

23

been involved in such issues since the 1970s. (A brief chronology can be found in Appendix C.) In 1999, because of IOM's previous work and its access to independent scientific experts, CDC and NIH began a year of discussions with IOM to develop the Immunization Safety Review project, which would address both emerging and existing vaccine safety issues.

The Immunization Safety Review Committee is responsible for examining a broad variety of immunization safety concerns. Committee members have expertise in pediatrics, neurology, immunology, internal medicine, infectious diseases, genetics, epidemiology, biostatistics, risk perception and communication, decision analysis, public health, nursing, and ethics. While all of the committee members share the view that immunization is generally beneficial, none of them has a vested interest in the specific immunization safety issues that come before the group. Additional discussion of the committee composition can be found in the Foreword, written by Dr. Harvey Fineberg, President of the IOM.

The committee is charged with examining up to three immunization safety hypotheses each year during the three-year study period (2001–2003). These hypotheses are selected by the Interagency Vaccine Group (IAVG), whose members represent several units of the Department of Health and Human Services: the CDC's National Vaccine Program Office, National Immunization Program, and National Center for Infectious Diseases; the NIH's National Institute of Allergy and Infectious Diseases; the Food and Drug Administration; the Health Resources and Services Administration's National Vaccine Injury Compensation Program; and the Centers for Medicare and Medicaid Services (formerly the Health Care Financing Administration). The IAVG includes representation from the Department of Defense and the Agency for International Development as well.

For each topic, the Immunization Safety Review Committee reviews relevant literature and submissions by interested parties, holds an open scientific meeting, and directly follows the open meeting with a 1- to 2-day closed meeting to formulate its conclusions and recommendations. The committee's findings are released to the public in a brief consensus report 60 to 90 days after its meeting.

The committee is charged with assessing both the scientific evidence regarding the hypotheses under review and the significance of the issues for society.

- The *scientific* assessment has two components: (1) an examination of the epidemiologic and clinical evidence regarding a possible *causal relationship* between exposure to the vaccine and the adverse event; and (2) an examination of theory and experimental or observational evidence from *in vitro*, animal, or human studies regarding *biological mechanisms* that might be relevant to the hypothesis.
- The *significance* assessment addresses such considerations as the burden of the health risks associated with both the vaccine-preventable disease and the adverse event. Other considerations may include the perceived intensity of public or professional concern, or the feasibility of additional research to help resolve scientific uncertainty regarding causality.

The findings of the scientific and significance assessments provide the basis for the committee's recommendations regarding the public health response to the issue. In particular, the committee addresses any needs for a review of immunization policy, for current and future research, and for effective communication strategies. See Figure 1 for a schematic representation of the committee's charge.

THE STUDY PROCESS

The committee held an initial organizational meeting in January 2001. CDC and NIH presented the committee's charge at the meeting, and the committee then conducted a general review of immunization safety concerns. At this initial meeting, the committee also determined the basic methodology to be used for assessing causality in the hypotheses to be considered at subsequent meetings. A website (www.iom.edu/imsafety) and a listserv were created to provide public access to information about the committee's work and to facilitate communication with the committee. The conclusions and recommendations of the committee's reports thus far (see Box 1) are summarized in Appendix A.

For its evaluation of the question concerning influenza vaccines and neurological complications, the committee held an open scientific meeting in March 2003 (see Appendix B) to hear presentations on issues germane to the topic. These presentations are available in electronic form (audio files and slides) on the project website (www.iom.edu/imsafety). In addition, the committee reviewed an extensive collection of material, primarily from the published, peer-reviewed scientific and medical literature. A list of the materials reviewed by the committee, including many items not cited in this report, can be found on the project's website.

THE FRAMEWORK FOR SCIENTIFIC ASSESSMENT

Causality

The Immunization Safety Review Committee has adopted the framework for assessing causality developed by previous IOM committees (IOM, 1991; 1994a,b) convened under the congressional mandate of P.L. 99-660 to address questions of immunization safety. The categories of causal conclusions used by the committee are as follows:

1. No evidence
2. Evidence is inadequate to accept or reject a causal relationship
3. Evidence favors rejection of a causal relationship
4. Evidence favors acceptance of a causal relationship
5. Evidence establishes a causal relationship.

26

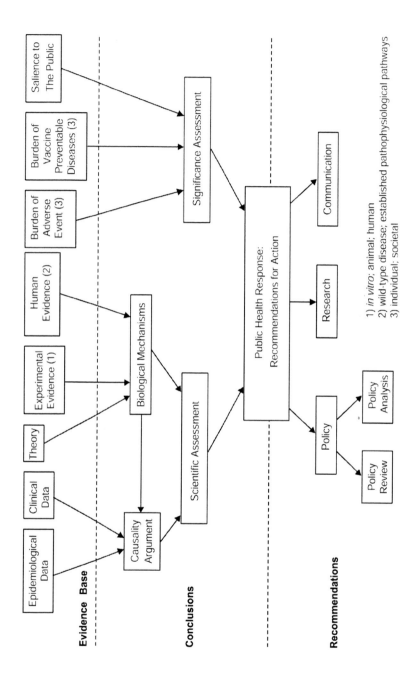

FIGURE 1 Committee charge.

BOX 1
Previous Reports of the Immunization Safety Review Committee

Immunization Safety Review: Measles-Mumps-Rubella Vaccine and Autism (IOM, 2001a)

Immunization Safety Review: Thimerosal-Containing Vaccines and Neuro-developmental Disorders (IOM, 2001b)

Immunization Safety Review: Multiple Immunizations and Immune Dysfunction (IOM, 2002b)

Immunization Safety Review: Hepatitis B Vaccine and Demyelinating Neurological Disorders (IOM, 2002a)

Immunization Safety Review: SV40 Contamination of Polio Vaccine and Cancer (IOM, 2002c)

Immunization Safety Review: Vaccinations and Sudden Unexpected Death in Infancy (IOM, 2003)

Assessments begin from a position of neutrality regarding the specific immunization safety hypothesis under review. That is, there is no presumption that a specific vaccine (or vaccine component) does or does not cause the adverse event in question. The weight of the available clinical and epidemiologic evidence determines whether it is possible to shift from that neutral position to a finding for causality ("the evidence favors acceptance of a causal relationship") or against causality ("the evidence favors rejection of a causal relationship"). The committee does not conclude that the vaccine does not cause the adverse event merely if the evidence is inadequate to support causality. Instead, it maintains a neutral position, concluding that the "evidence is inadequate to accept or reject a causal relationship."

Although no firm rules establish the amount of evidence or the quality of the evidence required to support a specific category of causality conclusion, the committee uses standard epidemiologic criteria to guide its decisions. The most definitive category is "establishes causality," which is reserved for those relationships in which the causal link is unequivocal, as with the oral polio vaccine and vaccine-associated paralytic polio or with anaphylactic reactions to vaccine administration (IOM 1991; 1994a). The next category, "favors acceptance" of a causal relationship, reflects evidence that is strong and generally convincing, although not firm enough to be described as unequivocal or established. "Favors rejection" is the strongest category in the negative direction. (The category of "establishes no causal relationship" is *not* used because it is virtually impossible to prove the absence of a relationship with the same surety that is possible in establishing the presence of one.)

If the evidence is not reasonably convincing either in support of or against causality, the category "inadequate to accept or reject a causal relationship" is used. Evidence that is sparse, conflicting, of weak quality, or merely suggestive—whether toward or away from causality—falls into this category. Under these circumstances, some authors of similar assessments use phrases such as "the evidence does not presently support a causal association." The committee believes, however, that such language does not make the important distinction between evidence indicating that a relationship does not exist (category 3) and evidence that is indeterminate with regard to causality (category 2).

The category of "no evidence" is reserved for those cases in which there is a complete absence of clinical or epidemiologic evidence.

The sources of evidence considered by the committee in its assessment of causality include epidemiologic and clinical studies directly addressing the question at hand. That is, the data are specifically related to the effects of the vaccine(s) under review and the adverse health outcome(s) under review—in this report, the effects of influenza vaccination on the risk of neurological complications.

Epidemiologic studies carry the most weight in a causality assessment. These studies measure health-related exposures and outcomes in a defined set of subjects and use that information to make inferences about the nature and strength of associations between such exposures and outcomes in the overall population from which the study sample was drawn. Epidemiologic studies can be categorized as observational or experimental (clinical trial) and as uncontrolled (descriptive) or controlled (analytic). Among the various study designs, experimental studies generally have the advantage of random assignment to exposures and are therefore the most influential in assessing causality. Uncontrolled observational studies are important but are generally considered less definitive than controlled studies. In uncontrolled observational studies, where observations are made over time, confounding factors such as changing case definitions or improving case detection may affect the apparent incidence and prevalence of the adverse outcomes studied.

Case reports and case series are generally inadequate by themselves to establish causality. Despite the limitations of case reports, the causality argument for at least one vaccine-related adverse event (the relationship between vaccines containing tetanus toxoid and Guillain-Barré syndrome) was strengthened most by a single, well-documented case report on recurrence of the adverse event following re-administration of the vaccine, a situation referred to as a "rechallenge" (IOM, 1994a).

Biological Mechanisms

The committee's causality assessments must be guided by an understanding of relevant biological processes. Therefore the committee's scientific assessment includes consideration of biological mechanisms[1] by which immunizations might cause an adverse event. The evidence reviewed comes from human, animal, and *in vitro* studies of biological or pathophysiological processes relevant to the question before the committee.

When convincing statistical or clinical evidence of causality is available, biological data add support. But this committee is often faced with circumstances in which the epidemiologic evidence is judged inadequate to accept or reject a causal association between a vaccine exposure and an adverse event of concern. It is then left with the task of examining proposed or conceivable biological mechanisms that might be operating *if* an epidemiologically sound association could be shown between a vaccine exposure and an adverse event. The biological data alone cannot be invoked as proof of causality, however.

The committee has established three general categories of evidence on biological mechanisms:

1. *Theoretical.* A reasonable mechanism can be hypothesized that is commensurate with scientific knowledge and does not contradict known physical and biological principles, but has not been demonstrated in whole or in part in humans or animal models. Postulated mechanisms by which a vaccine might cause a specific adverse event but for which no coherent theory exists would not qualify for this category. Thus, "theoretical" is not a default category, but one that requires thoughtful and biologically meaningful suppositions.

2. *Experimental.* A mechanism can be shown to operate in *in vitro* systems, animals, or humans. But experimental evidence often describes mechanisms that represent only a portion of the pathological process required for expression of disease. Showing that multiple portions of a process operate in reasonable experimental models strengthens the case that the mechanisms could possibly result in disease in humans.

Some experimental evidence is derived under highly contrived conditions. For example, achieving the results of interest may require extensive manipulation of the genetics of an animal system, or *in vivo* or *in vitro* exposures to a vaccine antigen that are extreme in terms of dose, route, or duration. Other experimental evidence is derived under less contrived conditions. For example, a compelling animal or *in vitro* model might demonstrate a pathologic process analogous to human disease when a vaccine antigen is administered under conditions similar to human use. Experimental evidence can also come from studies in humans. In any case, biological evidence is distinct from the epidemiologic evidence obtained from randomized controlled trials and other population-based studies that are the basis for the causality assessment.

---

[1]For a discussion of the evolution of the terminology concerning biological mechanisms, see the committee's earlier reports (IOM, 2001a,b, 2002a,b).

3. *Evidence that the mechanism results in known disease in humans.* For example, the wild-type infection causes the adverse health outcome associated with the vaccine, or another vaccine has been demonstrated to cause the same adverse outcome by the same or a similar mechanism. Data from population-based studies of the risk of adverse outcomes following vaccination constitute evidence regarding causality, not biological mechanisms.

If the committee identifies evidence of biological mechanisms that could be operating, it offers a summary judgment of that body of evidence as weak, moderate, or strong. Although the committee tends to judge biological evidence in humans as "stronger" than biological evidence from highly contrived animal models or *in vitro* systems, the summary judgment of the strength of the evidence also depends on the quantity (e.g., number of studies or number of subjects in a study) and quality (e.g., the nature of the experimental system or study design) of the evidence. Obviously, the conclusions drawn from this review depend both on the specific data and scientific judgment. To ensure that its own summary judgment is defensible, the committee aims to be as explicit as possible regarding the strengths and limitations of the biological data.

The committee's examination of biological mechanisms reflects its opinion that available information on possible biological explanations for a relationship between immunization and an adverse event should influence the design of epidemiologic studies and analyses. Similarly, the consideration of confounders and effect modifiers is essential in epidemiologic studies and depends on an understanding of the biological phenomena that could underlie or explain the observed statistical relationship. The identification of sound biological mechanisms can also guide the development of an appropriate research agenda and aid policymakers, who frequently must make decisions without having definitive information regarding causality.

In addition, investigating and understanding possible biological mechanisms is often of value even if the available epidemiologic evidence suggests the absence of a causal association. A review of biological data could give support to the negative causality assessment, for example, or it could prompt a reconsideration or further investigation of the epidemiologic findings. If new epidemiologic studies were to question the existing causality assessment, the biological data could gain prominence in the new assessments.

Published and Unpublished Data

Published reports carry the most weight in the committee's assessment because their methods and findings are laid out in enough detail to be assessed. Furthermore, those published works that undergo a rigorous peer review are subject to comment and criticism by the entire scientific community. In general, the committee cannot rely heavily on unpublished data in making its scientific assessments (regarding either causality or biological mechanisms) because they usually lack the commentary and criticism provided by peer review and must therefore be interpreted with caution. The committee also relies on editorial and peer-review procedures to ensure the disclosure of potential conflicts of interest that might be related to sources of funding of the research studies. The committee does not investigate the sources of funding of the published research reports it reviews, nor do funding sources influence the committee's interpretation of the evidence.

Unpublished data and other reports that have not undergone peer review do have value, however, and are often considered by the committee. They might be used, for example, in support of a body of published, peer-reviewed literature with similar findings. If the committee concluded that the unpublished data were well described, had been obtained using sound methodology, and presented very clear results, the committee could report, with sufficient caveats in the discussion, how the unpublished data fit with the entire body of published literature. Only in extraordinary circumstances, however, could an unpublished study refute a body of published literature.

The Immunization Safety Review Committee's scope of work includes consideration of clinical topics for which high-quality experimental studies are rarely available. Although many other panels making clinical recommendations using evidence-based methods are able to require that randomized trials be available to reach strong conclusions, the IOM committee was convened specifically to assess topics that are of immediate concern yet for which data of any kind may just be emerging. Given the unique nature of this project, therefore, the committee deemed it important to review and consider as much information as possible, including unpublished reports. The committee does not perform primary or secondary analyses of unpublished data, however. In reviewing unpublished material, the committee applies generally accepted standards for assessing the quality of scientific evidence, as described above. (All unpublished data reviewed by the committee and cited in this report are available—in the form reviewed by the committee—through the public access files of the National Academies. Information about the public access files is available at 202-334-3543 or www.national-academies.org/publicaccess.)

UNDER REVIEW:
INFLUENZA VACCINES AND NEUROLOGICAL COMPLICATIONS

The Immunization Safety Review Committee was asked to examine the hypothesis that a causal relationship might exist between receipt of influenza vaccines and neurological complications. In the United States, concern about such adverse neurological events is most prominently linked to cases of Guillain-

Barré syndrome (GBS) that occurred following the administration of influenza vaccine to between 40-45 million people in the 1976 National Influenza Immunization Program (CDC, 2003c; Langmuir et al., 1984).

This federally funded immunization program was aimed at averting the possibility of an outbreak of a type of influenza—"swine flu"—thought to be related to the virus that caused a massive global epidemic in 1918–1919. Although production of a vaccine was slowed by technical problems as well as by negotiations between the government and manufacturers over the purchase contracts and liability protections, ultimately, the production, distribution, and administration of the swine influenza vaccine was successfully implemented. However, the vaccination program was halted in December 1976 when no pandemic was evident and after more than 500 cases of GBS were reported among U.S. vaccinees, which appeared to be associated with the vaccine (Kitch et al., 1999).

When a CDC-sponsored study showed a statistically significant association between vaccination and an increase in the risk of GBS during the 10 weeks following vaccination, the federal government agreed to accept liability for all cases of GBS with onset falling within this period (Kitch et al., 1999). More than $90 million was paid by the government to cover claims on these cases. The large scale of the program and the administration of vaccine within a narrow time window offered an opportunity to identify a vaccine-related event as rare as GBS. The detection of such a rare and unexpected event such as the association of the vaccine with GBS was facilitated by the large number of doses of vaccine administered in a narrow time window. The program also demonstrated the role of resource-intensive surveillance for rare adverse events and the significance of liability concerns, both for the government and vaccine manufacturers.

The committee's review of the evidence concerning risks that might be associated with influenza vaccines had to take into account a distinctive feature of the vaccine: its formulation changes from year to year to reflect changes in the strains of influenza virus circulating in the population. As a result, the question before the committee actually concerns many different influenza vaccines rather than a single, consistent product used over many years. In terms of the neurological outcomes of concern, GBS is the most widely cited. Other outcomes considered by the committee are multiple sclerosis (MS) and optic neuritis. Key features of influenza, influenza viruses, and influenza vaccines are described below, followed by brief overviews of these outcomes.

Influenza and Influenza Vaccines

Influenza

Influenza is an acute and highly contagious viral respiratory disease that occurs worldwide. Up to 20 percent of the population may be infected in a single year (Palese and Garcia-Sastre, 2002). Although some infections are subclinical, influenza is responsible for substantial morbidity and mortality. The elderly, young children, and persons with chronic cardiac or pulmonary diseases are generally at greatest risk for fatal complications (Dolin, 2001). In the United States alone, the disease is now estimated to contribute to an average of 36,000 deaths each year, a toll that has risen as the population has aged (Thompson et al., 2003).

The incidence of influenza peaks during the winter months in temperate zones, but infections occur year-round in the tropics (Dolin, 2001). The extent and severity of influenza infections can vary widely from year to year. The disease frequently reaches epidemic levels and periodically becomes pandemic— referring to high levels of infection worldwide that are not necessarily associated with an unusually severe form of the disease (Kilbourne and Arden, 1999). The 1918–1919 pandemic, however, resulted in the deaths of an estimated 500,000 persons in the United States and 20 to 50 million persons worldwide, including large numbers of young adults (CDC, 2002a).

The influenza viruses infect the respiratory epithelium. Onset of illness is often abrupt, with systemic symptoms that include fever, chills, headache, myalgias and respiratory signs such as cough and sore throat. In uncomplicated cases, acute illness typically resolves over 2 to 5 days. Recovery may be complete within a week, but some patients experience persistent weakness or lassitude (Dolin, 2001). Treatment generally consists of symptomatic therapy, such as acetaminophen for headache, myalgia or fever. Antiviral drugs may also be effective if therapy is started within 48 hours of the onset of illness (Dolin, 2001).

Many of the influenza-related deaths result from complications, the most common being secondary bacterial pneumonia (e.g., *Streptococcus pneumoniae, Haemophilus influenzae,* or *Staphylococcus aureus*). Primary viral pneumonia is less common but has a high fatality rate. Influenza can also exacerbate chronic pulmonary conditions or contribute to a general deterioration in cardiac or pulmonary function, especially in the elderly or persons with chronic illness. Other complications sometimes seen include myositis, rhabdomyolysis, and myoglobinuria (Dolin, 2001; Hilleman, 2002).

A temporal association between neurological complications such as encephalitis, transverse myelitis, and GBS has also been reported (Dolin, 2001). Encephalitis/encephalopathy has been reported as a complication primarily of influenza type A (H3N2) infections in Japanese children, although a causal relationship has not been proven (Morishima et al., 2002; Sugaya, 2002). Others have reported smaller numbers of cases of encephalitis associated with influenza B infections in children in the United States and elsewhere (Newland et al., 2003). The CDC (2003a) has recently requested information to try to identify additional cases of acute encephalopathy that may have occurred in children with influenza since January 1998.

Factors that have been proposed as possibly accounting for the complications observed in the Japanese children include genetic characteristics in the Japanese population, infection with a particularly virulent viral strain, and regional differences in diagnostic criteria (Morishima et al., 2002; Sugaya, 2002; Yoshikawa et al., 2001). Although the Japanese cases are described as distinct from Reye's syndrome, which is closely associated with the administration of aspirin in viral infections, the non-aspirin antipyretics (e.g., diclofenac sodium) used in Japan are being studied to clarify whether they might be associated with increased risk for encephalitis/encephalopathy (Morishima et al., 2002).

Influenza Viruses

Influenza viruses are members of the family Orthomyxoviridae. Three forms of the virus—referred to as types A, B, and C—are known to infect humans. The B and C viruses circulate exclusively in humans, with type C producing little illness. Type A viruses, however, circulate not only in humans but also in wild aquatic birds, their natural reservoir. In addition, the type A viruses infect other birds and several species of mammals.

Influenza A viruses are subtyped based on antigenic characteristics of their spike-like surface glycoproteins hemagglutinin (HA) and neuraminidase (NA) (Dolin, 2001). There are 15 known subtypes of HA and 9 subtypes of NA in influenza A viruses (Steinhauer and Skehel, 2002). All of these subtypes are found in wild aquatic birds. Various subtypes circulate in other birds and mammals as well. To date, only H1N1, H2N2, and H3N2 are known to circulate extensively in humans, although other subtypes are found sporadically. Influenza B and C viruses also carry HA and NA surface antigens, but they are not given subtype designations. Individual strains of all three types of influenza virus have unique designations that reflect the location and year of the identified strain. For example, the type A swine influenza virus that prompted the 1976 immunization program in the United States is referred to as A/New Jersey/76 (H1N1).

Immunity to influenza depends on the formation of antibodies to the glycoprotein surface antigens HA and NA (Dolin, 2001; Hilleman, 2002). However, influenza viruses of types A and B are successful in evading pre-existing immunity from prior infections or vaccination because HA and NA continuously evolve (Dolin, 2001; CDC, 2002a). The influenza A and B virus genomes consists of eight strands of negative-sense RNA that encode 10 viral proteins (see Table 1) (Dolin, 2001; Hilleman, 2002; Steinhauer and Skehel, 2002; Ziegler and Cox, 1999). Replication of the genetic material is error-prone and there is no proof-reading mechanism, allowing for the accumulation of point mutations. Such mutations in the genes encoding the surface antigens lead to what is called antigenic drift.

The influenza A virus is also subject to antigenic shift—a major change in the HA or NA antigens (e.g., from H1 to H2 or N1 to N2). Antigenic shift is thought to be the result of gene reassortments between different virus strains, including strains circulating in animals. Pigs have been proposed as a potential host for reassortment because replication of both human and avian viruses can

TABLE 1 Components and Products of the Influenza A Virus Genome

RNA segment	Gene product	Role
1	PB-2	Subunits of viral polymerase
2	PB-1	
3	PA	
4	Hemagglutinin (HA)	Receptor binding, fusion of viral envelope to cell membrane
5	Nucleoprotein (NP)	Encapsidates RNA segments
6	Neuraminidase (NA)	Cleaves host cell sialic acid, prevents viral aggregation, facilitates release of progeny virus
7	Matrix proteins	
	M1	Interacts with genome, assists in viral assembly
	M2	Ion channel, controls pH during HA synthesis and virion uncoating
8	Nonstructural (NS) proteins	
	NS1	Regulation of mRNA splicing and translation, interferon antagonist.
	NS2 or NEP	Nuclear export of viral RNA, viral assembly

SOURCE: Adapted from Hilleman, 2002.

TABLE 2 Antigenic Shifts in Influenza A Subtypes During the 20th Century

Year	Viral Subtype	Associated Health Impact (in the U.S.)
1918	H1N1	Severe—500,000 deaths
1957	H2N2	Severe—70,00 deaths
1968	H3N2	Moderate—34,000 deaths
1977	H1N1	Mild

SOURCE: Adapted from CDC, 2002a.

occur in pigs. Antigenic shift is associated with pandemic infection. The four antigenic shifts that occurred during the 20th century are listed in Table 2. Since 1977, H3N2 and H1N1 subtypes have been co-circulating in humans. Antigenic drift occurs often, leading the need for annual influenza vaccination. Antigenic shift occurs less frequently and is associated with changes in morbidity and mortality.

Influenza Vaccines

Vaccination is the primary means of reducing the impact of influenza, either by preventing illness or reducing its severity. Estimates of vaccination coverage for 2001 were 67 percent for adults aged 65 years or older and 35 percent for adults aged 50–64 years. Estimates from 2000 showed that vaccination coverage was 29 percent among adults aged 18–64 years who had high-risk health conditions. Coverage among children for whom influenza vaccination is recommended are said to be low, but systematic data are not readily available (CDC, 2003d).

The Advisory Committee on Immunization Practices (ACIP) currently recommends influenza vaccination for persons 6 months of age and older who are at increased risk for complications of influenza, all persons 50 to 64 years old, and health care workers and others who can transmit influenza to those at high risk for complications (CDC, 2003d). Persons considered to be at high risk for complications from influenza include persons aged 65 years or older; residents of nursing homes and chronic care facilities; children and adults with chronic lung, heart, kidney, metabolic, or immune system disorders; and women who will be in the second or third trimester of pregnancy during influenza season. ACIP also encourages that children aged 6-23 months receive the influenza vaccine. A recommendation for universal routine influenza immunization in that age group may be made in the near future (CDC, 2003d).

The majority of vaccines currently approved for use in the United States are inactivated ("killed virus") influenza vaccines.[2] These vaccines can be formulated as whole virus or "split" (subvirion or purified surface antigen) products. Only split-virus vaccines are available in the United States. In addition to inactivated vaccines, attenuated live-virus vaccines are used in some other countries (Wareing and Tannock, 2001). A live attenuated intranasal influenza vaccine was approved by the FDA in June 2003 for use in the United States in healthy individuals aged 5-49 years (DHHS, 2003). Current vaccines are trivalent, produced using strains of influenza A(H1N1), influenza A(H3N2), and influenza B viruses. Because of the continuing antigenic changes in these viruses, new influenza vaccines are formulated each year based on information on the viral strains that circulated during the previous season or are circulating at the time in other parts of the world. The effectiveness of influenza vaccines depends, in part, on the match between the viral strains used to produce them and the strains that actually circulate in the subsequent influenza season. If the viral strains used to produce the vaccine are closely matched to the viral strains circulating during the influenza season, vaccination may prevent illness (although not necessarily infection)

---

[2]Inactivated influenza vaccines licensed for use in the United States for the 2002 influenza season included FluShield (Wyeth Lederle); Fluvirin (Evans Vaccines, Ltd.); and Fluzone (Aventis Pasteur). As of November 2002, Wyeth ceased producing FlueShield. The live attenuated vaccine FluMist is manufactured by MedImmune Vaccines, Inc and marketed by Wyeth Vaccines.

in 70 to 90 percent of healthy children as young as 6 months of age and healthy adults under age 65. (CDC, 2002b).

The World Health Organization coordinates a system of worldwide surveillance of influenza infection and recommends viral strains to be used in each year's vaccines. CDC collaborates in this surveillance activity and is responsible for monitoring influenza morbidity and mortality in the United States. Every year between January and March, FDA and CDC identify the strains that are recommended for use in formulating the vaccine for the coming influenza season in the United States. Ideally, influenza vaccine is ready for distribution in time for vaccination campaigns to begin in the fall before the start of influenza season.

Manufacturers begin preparations for vaccine production while the strain selection is being completed. The FDA prepares the specific reference virus stock for manufacturers, who then incorporate the HA and NA genetic components from the FDA reference viruses into their proprietary, high-yield seed virus strains. Virus for the vaccines is cultivated in embryonated chicken eggs and purified from the allantoic fluid by zonal centrifugation or chromatography. The purified live virus is inactivated (killed) with formalin or beta-propiolactone. To prepare split-virus vaccines, the killed virus is treated with organic solvents or detergents. Split-virus vaccines prepared with solvents, the subvirion vaccines, contain all the viral structural proteins and portions of the viral membrane. Virus treated with detergent is used to produce subunit or purified surface antigen vaccines, which are enriched for HA and NA and contain only residual internal structural proteins. Thimerosal is used as a preservative in vaccines distributed in multi-dose vials and in some single-dose syringes. A limited supply of preservative-free vaccine is also prepared as single dose pre-filled syringes (although preservative is not included in the final formulation, these preparations do contain a trace amount of thimerosal from the manufacturing process) (CDC, 2003d).

Subvirion and purified antigen influenza vaccines are similar in immunogenicity and are less reactogenic than whole-virus preparations, especially in children (Beyer et al., 1998; Kilbourne and Arden, 1999). Nevertheless, because influenza vaccines are produced in eggs and may contain residual egg protein, special caution has to be exercised in giving them to individuals who are allergic to egg products (Kilbourne and Arden, 1999).

Summarized in Box 2 are similarities and differences among influenza vaccines in terms of the manufacturing processes used and the content of the resulting vaccine. The influenza vaccines that were used in the 1976 swine influenza vaccination program were produced using similar methods, except that both whole-cell and subunit vaccines were manufactured. Some of the vaccine produced in 1976 was monovalent, using only the influenza A(H1N1) subtype, and some was bivalent, incorporating both the A(H1N1) and A(H3N2) subtypes. The timeline for production of swine flu vaccine was compressed, compared with other years, with vaccination beginning less than eight months after the strain was first identified.

BOX 2
Similarities and Differences in the Manufacturing and Content of Influenza Vaccines Used in the United States[1]

	Similarities	Differences
Manufacturing	• Virus cultured in embryonated chicken eggs • Influenza reference virus provided by FDA • Purification steps to remove nonviral (egg) materials and chemicals • Chemical inactivation • Sterile, but with some residual endotoxin • Preservative	• Proprietary chicken flocks • Proprietary seed viruses • Process differences: zonal centrifugation vs. chromatography, disrupting agent (detergents and lipid solvents, e.g., ether, Triton X 100)
Content	• Hemagglutinins standardized to a minimum of 15 micrograms per strain per dose • Limits for maximum endotoxin content • Limits for chemical excipients (disrupting agents and inactivating agents)	• Total protein content • Residual viral proteins (NA, NP, M) • Endotoxin content • Formalin vs. beta propiolactone • Thimerosal content • Adjuvants (none used in U.S. licensed vaccines)

[1]From 1990 to 2003, influenza vaccines used in the United States were manufacturered by Connaught (Aventis Pasteur), Swiftwater, PA, USA; Evans Vaccines, Liverpool, England; Wyeth Vaccines, Marietta, PA, USA (ceased 2002); and Parke-Davis (Parkedale), Rochester, MI (ceased 2000).
SOURCE: Adapted from Levandowski, 2003.

Adverse Neurological Events

The adverse events considered in this report—GBS, MS, and optic neuritis—are primarily diseases involving demyelination of nerve cell axons in either the central (CNS) or peripheral (PNS) nervous systems. Myelin, a principal component of what is referred to as the white matter of the nervous system, normally surrounds the axons of many nerve cells, providing protection and contributing to the transmission of signals through the nervous system. In the CNS (the brain, spinal cord, and optic nerves), myelin is synthesized by oligodendrocytes; in the

PNS, it is synthesized by Schwann cells. Oligodendrocytes typically ensheath several axonal processes, and the expression of myelin genes by the oligodendrocytes appears to depend on the presence of astrocytes. In contrast, the external cell membrane of each Schwann cell surrounds a single axon, and the expression of myelin genes is regulated by contact between the axon and the myelinating Schwann cell.

Demyelination occurs when the sheaths around nerve cell axons are damaged by inflammatory or other injurious processes, including autoimmune mechanisms. The damage to the myelin sheath exposes the axon to the risk of injury and interferes with the transmission of nerve impulses. Remyelination can occur and is more effective in the PNS than in the CNS. This difference is probably related to the respective tissue environments, with peripheral nerves exposed to growth factors and other mediators that are not present in or are less accessible to the CNS (Waubant and Stuve, 2002).

Several other neurological complications have been reported following receipt of influenza vaccines, including transverse myelitis, hypoglossal nerve paralysis, hemiparesis, meningoencephalitic syndrome, and ADEM (acute disseminated encephalomyelitis). The committee found no systematic study of their possible association with influenza vaccines, and therefore these conditions have not been described here.

Guillain-Barré Syndrome

GBS is an acute, immune-mediated paralytic disorder of the peripheral nervous system. It is the most common cause of acute flaccid paralysis in the post-polio era. Estimates of the annual incidence of GBS range from 0.4 to 4.0 cases per 100,000 population, with most studies pointing to a level of from 1 to 2 cases per 100,000 (Hughes and Rees, 1997; Magira et al., 2003). GBS occurs throughout the year, and in the United States the condition is more likely to occur in adults than in children (Asbury, 2000).

About two-thirds of GBS cases occur several days or weeks after an infectious event (Hughes and Rees, 1997), commonly a diarrheal illness or a virus-like upper-respiratory infection. Viral pathogens associated with GBS include human immunodeficiency virus, Epstein-Barr virus, and cytomegalovirus. Other risk factors for the development of GBS appear to include surgery and malignant disorders, especially lymphomas (IOM, 1994a).

From 20 percent to 40 percent of all GBS cases are associated with *Campylobacter jejuni* infections (Buzby et al., 1997). Often present in the sera of these patients are autoreactive antibodies to gangliosides. Gangliosides are a type of glycolipid found throughout the body, with high concentrations in nervous system tissue (Ledeen, 1985). More than 100 different forms of ganglioside are known. It is hypothesized that the antiganglioside antibodies found in some GBS patients may be induced as a result of molecular mimicry between peripheral nerve gangliosides and structurally similar lipopolysaccharides of *C. jejuni* (Moran and Prendergast, 2001; Nachamkin, 2002; Sheikh et al., 1998). (Molecular mimicry is discussed further in the review of evidence regarding biological mechanisms.)

Exposure to certain vaccines has also been associated with an increased risk of GBS. One example is the Semple rabies vaccines (used outside the United States) that were produced from nerve tissue of infected animals (Plotkin et al., 1995). Other examples include tetanus toxoid containing vaccines and oral polio vaccine. A previous IOM committee concluded that the evidence favored acceptance of a causal relation with receipt of those vaccines and GBS (IOM, 1994a). However, a study (Rantala et al., 1994) published after the release of that IOM report suggests to some that the relationship with the oral polio vaccine is not, in fact, causal (Sutter et al., 1999). The potential association between GBS and influenza vaccines, most notably the 1976 swine influenza vaccines, has been widely studied and is the principle focus of this report.

Until recently, GBS had been considered synonymous with acute inflammatory demyelinating polyradiculoneuropathy (AIDP), but research has shown that GBS is really a group of heterogenous but related disorders (see Box 3). In addition to the demyelinating AIDP, there are two axonal forms—acute motor axonal neuropathy (AMAN) and acute motor sensory axonal neuropathy (AMSAN)—and the cranial nerve variant, Miller Fisher syndrome (MFS) (Asbury, 2000; Joseph and Tsao, 2002). More than 90 percent of GBS cases seen in the United States are considered to be AIDP (Asbury, 2000). For the purposes of this report's examination of evidence concerning GBS and influenza vaccines, GBS has been treated as a single entity.

The characteristic clinical feature of GBS is an acute, rapidly progressive, symmetrical weakness, with loss of deep tendon reflexes, possible tingling in the feet and hands, and muscle aches (myalgia). Classically, symptoms progress in an ascending fashion, affecting legs first, but weakness and paresthesias may occasionally appear first in the arm or face and progress in a descending fashion. The severity of the motor impairment can range from mild weakness to total paralysis, and the severity of the sensory symptoms from minimal numbness and tingling to severe pain. Facial, oculomotor, oropharyngeal, and respiratory muscles may also be involved, and some patients may require respiratory support.

The severity of clinical deficits typically peaks within the first 2 weeks of onset, but some deficits may continue to progress for 3 to 4 weeks. Approximately 85 percent of patients will return to normal functioning within 6 to 9 months, but some patients experience relapses or a prolonged disease course with residual neurological deficits (Asbury, 2000; Joseph and Tsao, 2002). The mortality rate is 3-5 percent, with patients succumbing to undetected respiratory failure, malfunction of the autonomic nervous system, or to complications of immobility such as sepsis or pulmonary embolism (Joseph and Tsao, 2002).

BOX 3
Characteristics of Subtypes of Guillain-Barré Syndrome

Acute inflammatory demyelinating polyradiculoneuropathy (AIDP)
AIDP is the predominant form of GBS in the United States and Europe, accounting for more than 90 percent of GBS cases. There are likely to be multiple target antigens on the surface of peripheral nervous system tissue, although the target is unknown in most cases. Antiganglioside antibodies, most commonly anti-GM_1, are present in some cases.

Acute motor axonal neuropathy (AMAN)
AMAN lacks features of demyelination and appears to be purely a motor disease. It is the predominant form of GBS in northern China, accounting for 65-80 percent of cases. A higher proportion of AMAN patients have antecedent *C. jejuni* infections than do AIDP patients. Antibodies to gangliosides GD_{1a} and GM_1 can be detected in patient sera.

Acute motor sensory axonal neuropathy (AMSAN)
AMSAM is an uncommon, axonal form of GBS. It is similar to AMAN but also affects the sensory nerves and dorsal roots.

Miller Fisher syndrome (MFS)
MFS, also called Fisher syndrome, is an uncommon, demyelinating form of GBS. Patients experience paralysis of eye muscles (opthalmoplegoia), ataxia, and loss of tendon reflexes. More than 90 percent of patients with MFS are positive for the antiganglioside antibody anti-GQ_{1b}.

SOURCE: Asbury, 2000; Sheikh et al., 1998; Winer, 2001; Griffin, 2003.

Diagnosis of GBS is based primarily on clinical evaluation (Joseph and Tsao, 2002). Diagnostic criteria have varied over time and were made more strict in the wake of the concern about GBS raised by the 1976 swine influenza vaccination program (Asbury, 2000). Laboratory evaluation of cerebrospinal fluid (CSF) demonstrates raised protein levels with relatively normal cell count. Electromyography (EMG) and nerve conduction studies are also done as confirmatory tests.

Patients with GBS require careful monitoring and good supportive care. Treatment with plasmapheresis (also called plasma exchange) is an effective means for relieving symptoms and shortening the time to recovery (Joseph and Tsao, 2002; Raphael et al., 2001). The benefit of plasmapheresis appears to come from removing circulating antibodies thought to aggravate GBS. Comparable benefits are obtained with intravenous immunoglobulin (IVIG) (Asbury, 2000;

Hughes et al., 2001). Either form of immunotherapy must be started within 3 weeks of the first symptoms to be beneficial (Asbury, 2000).

Multiple Sclerosis

MS affects between 250,000 and 350,000 people in the United States and is the most common inflammatory demyelinating disease of the CNS (Keegan and Noseworthy, 2002). Its incidence and manifestations vary within the population. The relapsing-remitting form, for example, occurs predominantly in females (~1.6:1) but follows a more severe clinical course in males (Noseworthy et al., 2000). The incidence of the disease is highest in persons between the ages of 20 and 40 years, but it is also diagnosed in children as young as 2 years and in older individuals. MS is more frequent in populations of Northern European origin than in other ethnic groups (IOM, 2001c). The prevalence of the disease is between 50 and 250 cases per 100,000 people in high-risk areas such as the Scandinavian countries or the northern United States, whereas it is less than 5 cases per 100,000 in Africa and Japan (Waubant and Stuve, 2002).

Clinically, MS is characterized by a variety of neurological signs and symptoms, reflecting the occurrence of inflammatory demyelinating lesions throughout the CNS. Common presenting symptoms include focal sensory deficits, focal weakness, a loss of vision, double vision, imbalance, and fatigue. Sexual impairment as well as urinary and bowel dysfunction may occur. Approximately 50 percent of patients with MS may display some degree of cognitive impairment and psychiatric symptoms. The severity of the disease can range from subclinical forms that are diagnosed only after death from other causes to hyperacute forms that lead to death within the first few months after disease onset. About 20 percent of patients have a "benign" form of the disease, with little accumulation of disability by 10 or more years after the onset of the disease. However, 50 percent of MS patients develop a significant limitation in their ability to walk and require assistance within 15 years (Noseworthy et al., 2000).

Four principal disease patterns have been identified (Lublin and Reingold, 1996). More than 80 percent of patients with MS initially experience a relapsing-remitting course, with clinical exacerbations of neurological symptoms that are followed by complete or partial recovery. Exacerbations can last from 1 day to several weeks. Incomplete recovery from relapses can result in accumulation of disability. Approximately 50 percent of patients with the relapsing-remitting form of MS will experience a more progressive course of the disease after 10 years. Patients with this secondary progressive course of MS experience a gradual worsening of their disability, with or without superimposed exacerbations. Another 10 percent to 15 percent of patients have primary progressive MS, a form associated with the gradual progression of symptoms from onset without exacerbation or remission. A very small proportion of patients (1 percent to 5 percent) experience a course called progressive relapsing MS, which is progressive from onset and includes a few superimposed exacerbations during the course of the disease.

The clinical diagnosis of MS requires evidence of recurrent episodes of clinical exacerbations (dissemination in time) that represent dysfunctions in different anatomic locations within the CNS (dissemination in space). The diagnosis is often established only after the second attack, with the clinical onset of the disease defined retrospectively as the first clinical attack. Biological changes detectable in neuroimaging studies can precede the first appearance of clinical symptoms, but the timing of the onset of those changes is difficult to establish. Relapses are defined by the clinical onset of new, recurrent, or worsening neurological symptoms related to CNS dysfunction that last for 24 or more hours in the absence of fever or infection.

The cause of MS remains elusive, but disease susceptibility appears to involve both genetic and environmental factors. Genetic factors are reflected in an increased risk of developing MS among family members of MS patients. Regional differences in the incidence of MS and in clinical disease patterns may reflect differences in the distribution of genetic risk factors. The possible role of environmental factors is indicated by several epidemiological studies that have suggested that individuals who migrate after age 15 from regions with a high prevalence of MS to regions with a low prevalence of the disease, or vice versa, carry their native risk for contracting MS (Alter et al., 1966; Kurtzke et al., 1970). This suggests that exposure to an environmental factor, possibly an infectious agent, during childhood is critical for the development of MS. Reports of localized "clusters" (defined areas of unexpectedly high prevalence) of MS also suggest that a transmissible agent may contribute to this illness (Waubant and Stuve, 2002). But other analyses point to confounding factors that leave the role of environmental exposures uncertain (Noseworthy et al., 2000).

Optic Neuritis

Optic neuritis is caused by an inflammation of the optic nerve, with lesions occurring behind the orbit but anterior to the optic chiasm (IOM, 1994a). Symptoms include rapid vision loss, pain associated with eye movement, dimmed vision, abnormal color vision, altered depth perception, and Uhthoff's phenomenon (visual loss associated with an increase in body temperature) (IOM, 2001c). Symptoms generally worsen during the first 3 to 7 days before improving (IOM, 2001c). The majority of cases resolve within a few weeks to months of onset.

Optic neuritis can occur as an isolated monophasic disease, or it may be a symptom of other demyelinating diseases such as acute disseminated encephalomyelitis (ADEM) or MS. Optic neuritis is frequently, though not always, followed by a diagnosis of MS. The risk of developing MS within 15 years of an episode of optic neuritis is estimated to range from 45 to 80 percent (Purvin, 1998).

SCIENTIFIC ASSESSMENT

Causality

To assess the issue of causality, the committee examined epidemiologic evidence regarding the possibility of an association between exposure to influenza vaccines and neurological complications. The three outcomes of GBS, MS, and optic neuritis were considered separately. For GBS, the large number of studies (using active surveillance data) concerning the 1976 swine influenza vaccines were distinguished from the studies of influenza vaccines used in subsequent years. For MS, the committee reviewed studies involving the 1976 vaccine together with studies of later vaccines. The only epidemiologic data on optic neuritis come from a study conducted in the 1990s. For other neurological complications that have been observed following influenza vaccination, only case reports were found.

Concluding the assessment of these outcomes is a brief review of reports regarding neurological complications following administration of influenza vaccines to children. Influenza vaccine is given primarily to adults, and most of the evidence reviewed by the committee applies to persons aged 18 years or older.

Guillain-Barré Syndrome

For its review of the epidemiologic evidence regarding a possible association between influenza vaccination and GBS, the committee separated studies concerning the vaccines administered during the 1976 National Influenza Immunization Program from studies concerning influenza vaccines administered in subsequent years. Most of the studies of the 1976 vaccines were based on data collected through a system of active GBS surveillance that was instituted near the end of the 1976 immunization program. The data for studies of the vaccines used in later years came from various sources, including active surveillance programs specifically developed to collect data on GBS. The committee reviewed studies that presented data for the nation as a whole and studies based on data for individual states or for military personnel.

The published literature also includes case reports of GBS after receipt of the swine influenza vaccine (Houff et al., 1977; Poser and Behan, 1982; Poser et al., 1978; Postic et al., 1980; Seyal et al., 1978) and after receipt of other influenza vaccines (Knight et al., 1984; Brooks and Reznik, 1980; Winer et al., 1984).

For the period since 1990, case reports on GBS occurring after influenza vaccination are available from the Vaccine Adverse Event Reporting System (VAERS). The committee concluded that reports to VAERS and other case reports submitted to the committee are uninformative with respect to causality, although they are useful for hypothesis generation. Case reports help describe the domain of concerns, but the data are usually uncorroborated clinical descriptions that are insufficient to permit meaningful comment or to contribute to a causality argument. The analytical value of data from VAERS and other passive surveillance systems is limited by such problems as underreporting, lack of detail, inconsistent diagnostic criteria, and inadequate denominator data (Ellenberg and Chen, 1997; Singleton et al., 1999).

Of potentially greater value in assessing causality are "challenge-rechallenge" reports regarding a person who received a vaccine (or drug or other challenge) more than once and reacted adversely with the same disorder each time. For a challenge-rechallenge case to weigh heavily in a causality assessment, there must be certainty that the diagnosis is correct and that alternative etiological factors have been excluded. At the end of the section on influenza vaccines administered since 1976, four cases from VAERS are reviewed to assess their possible contribution as rechallenge cases.

1976 Swine Influenza Vaccines

Controlled Observational Studies

United States: Initial Analyses. Expanding on the preliminary report by Langmuir (1979), Schonberger and colleagues (1979) examined the association between GBS and influenza vaccination during the 1976 National Influenza Immunization Program. They used data collected through March 1978 by an active surveillance system for GBS cases that was established shortly before the national immunization program ended in mid-December 1976. The surveillance system operated in 11 selected states during the period December 3–16, 1976, and in the rest of the country thereafter.

During the course of the surveillance period, several methods were used to identify GBS cases with onset between October 1, 1976, and January 31, 1977. Initially, state health departments contacted practicing neurologists to collect basic information on any GBS case. Reports were telephoned to CDC on a daily basis. Some states also contacted non-neurologist physicians or hospitals or resurveyed neurologists after January 1977. In some analyses, data from nine states were omitted because of declines in case ascertainment after December 18, 1976.

In early January 1977, CDC requested use of a standardized form to report case histories, including vaccination status, medical history, and other relevant information (such as, clinical and laboratory findings, antecedent events, date of onset of neurologic symptoms, history of vaccination, and other demographic information). The criteria defining GBS cases were (1) diagnosis by a physician, and (2) objective evidence of muscle involvement. When vaccination was reported, a copy of the vaccination consent form was requested. The form identified the type of vaccine received (e.g., monovalent or bivalent) and the manufacturer's lot number for the dose received.

In total, about 45 million people in the civilian population were vaccinated as part of the National Influenza Immunization Program. CDC estimated the number of vaccinations administered each week from data collected from the states, which reported total vaccinations on a weekly basis and vaccinations administered by age group and type of vaccine (monovalent or bivalent) on a monthly basis. Weekly reporting ended in December 1976; monthly reporting continued through June 1977, with most of the reports during 1977 being for vaccinations administered in 1976. Schonberger and colleagues adjusted the data to account for late reports. Data from three or four states were omitted from certain analyses because of reporting discrepancies. Estimates of the U.S. population by state and age as of July 1, 1976, were obtained from the Bureau of the Census.

Estimates were also made of the amount of vaccine, by manufacturer and lot number, that was administered in each state. The amount of each vaccine lot on hand in each state in 1977 was compared with the lot-specific amounts of vaccine distributed. Overall, health departments received about 100 million doses of influenza vaccines produced by four manufacturers.

A total of 1098 patients with GBS were reported to the CDC. Of these, 532 were considered vaccinated with the A/New Jersey/76 influenza vaccine prior to their GBS onset and 543 were not vaccinated. The 15 patients who received the vaccine after onset of GBS were considered unvaccinated. The vaccination status of eight GBS cases was unknown.

Schonberger and colleagues (1979) produced a descriptive analysis of the GBS trends during the swine influenza immunization program and made comparisons between the vaccinated and unvaccinated groups. In the unvaccinated population, the incidence of GBS was stable during the study period, whereas cases in the vaccinated population increased from October through December and peaked around December 18. By January, the attack rate in the vaccinated population was similar to that of the unvaccinated group. The average attack rate for unvaccinated cases over 17 years of age was 0.22 cases per million per week, which compares with rates of 2.8 and 3.5 per million per week in the second and third weeks, respectively, after vaccination. The authors reported a nonrandom pattern of GBS onset in the vaccinated population: 71 percent of vaccinated cases became ill during the first 4 weeks after vaccination, and 52 percent became ill during the second and third weeks after receipt of the vaccine.

Other differences between cases in the vaccinated and unvaccinated populations included a higher median age among the vaccinated (46 years compared to 34.5 years); a smaller percentage of cases under age 20 in the vaccinated group (3 percent versus 26.1 percent), and a lower percentage of males in the vaccinated group (46.5 percent versus 55.2 percent). The groups showed a statistically significant difference in the percentages of cases diagnosed by a neurologist (83.1 percent vaccinated, 89.1 percent unvaccinated), reporting sensory symptoms (89.5 percent vaccinated, 79.9 percent unvaccinated), reporting cranial nerve involvement (53.3 percent vaccinated, 45.1 percent unvaccinated), and reporting acute illness 4 weeks prior to onset (32.8 percent vaccinated, 61.8 percent unvaccinated). Other significant differences included the percentage of reports with elevated CSF proteins (82.3 percent vaccinated, 74.7 percent unvaccinated) and with chronic illness (45.1 percent vaccinated, 35.6 percent unvaccinated). The risk for GBS following vaccination was similar across the United States.

The authors calculated age-specific attack rates, attributable risks, and relative risks. Attack rates were based on the 6-week period after receipt of the vaccine. (The surveillance period allowed for a maximum interval of 6 weeks for persons vaccinated during the final days of the immunization program.) Relative risks were calculated by comparing the attack rates for the vaccinated with those for the unvaccinated, and attributable risk was calculated by multiplying the difference between the attack rates in the vaccinated and unvaccinated groups by 1.37 (i.e., the ratio of 6 weeks to the length of the average month in the study period). The relative risk for all ages was 9.2 (95% CI 8.2-10.3), and the relative risk for cases aged 18 years and older was 7.6 (95% CI 6.7-8.6). The attributable risk within 6 weeks after vaccination for each of these age groups was 8.8 per million vaccinees. The authors reported no significant differences in risk between the bivalent and monovalent vaccines or between the split- and whole-virus vaccines.

The authors concluded that the findings demonstrated an increased risk of GBS after swine influenza vaccination. Evidence included the nonrandom distribution of intervals between vaccination and GBS onset, the clustering of cases within the first 4 weeks after vaccination, and the lower proportion of cases with prior acute illness among the vaccinated. The authors also noted that one possible limitation was that no precise diagnostic criteria for GBS were used, but most of the cases were diagnosed by a neurologist and the differences in the clinical characteristics of the vaccinated and unvaccinated cases were not as great as differences in attack rates between the two groups.

In a separate report, Keenlyside and colleagues (1980) reviewed the 58 fatalities among the 1098 cases of GBS with onset between October 1, 1976, and January 31, 1977. Among the fatal cases, 32 had received a swine influenza vaccine. The overall case fatality rate of 5.3 percent was described as similar to the rate of 7 percent reported for an earlier 14-year period. Separate fatality rates for the vaccinated and unvaccinated cases were not presented. The authors reported that the mean interval from onset to death was significantly longer for vaccinated cases (56 days) than for unvaccinated (30 days), but they did not report statistical values. The differences between the vaccinated and unvaccinated cases in their history of prior acute or chronic illness were reported as not significant.

United States: Reanalysis. During litigation of damage claims related to the swine influenza vaccine, the reports by Langmuir (1979) and Schonberger and colleagues (1979) were criticized for lack of detail on the basic data analyzed and for the methods used to calculate risk (Langmuir et al., 1984). In response to a court order issued in 1981, Langmuir and colleagues (1984) reanalyzed the data on cases of GBS with onset between October 1, 1976, and January 31, 1977.

As the basis for their analysis, Langmuir and colleagues (1984) had one-page, computer-generated summaries for each of the 1098 cases in the analysis by Schonberger and colleagues (1979), computer line-listings of the data for these cases, and data on the estimated number of vaccinations administered each week during the immunization program. The authors had no access to the original reports compiled by CDC. They also were not permitted to interview personnel who had been involved in the National Influenza Immunization Program. However, one former CDC staff member from the immunization program was responsible for preparing the computerized data reviewed for the study.

Langmuir and colleagues (1984) excluded from their analysis 33 cases with insufficient data and 121 cases who were less than 18 years of age. (Adults were the primary target population for the vaccine.) The clinical data for the remaining 944 cases were reviewed, and cases were classified by extent of the motor involvement. Cases with "extensive" motor involvement (n = 580) had paresis or paralysis of extremities plus involvement of the trunk or cranial muscles, with or without respiratory impairment. Cases with "limited" motor involvement (n = 242) had paresis or paralysis of only the extremities (either three to four or one to two extremities). The remaining cases (n = 122) were classified as "insufficient" because key clinical data were missing or conflicting.

The clinical data were reviewed without access to information on vaccination status. Of the 944 cases, 504 had been vaccinated and 440 were unvaccinated. Langmuir and colleagues concluded that the data showed no difference between the vaccinated and unvaccinated cases in the adequacy of the clinical data reported. There was an indication, however, that ascertainment of new GBS cases in unvaccinated persons declined after the immunization program ended.

Estimates were made of the number of vaccinations administered each week from October 1, 1976, through December 16, 1976. Vaccination data that had been collected each week in conjunction with the immunization program were compared with vaccination reports from weekly rounds of the National Health Survey. The survey data were considered less prone to reporting lags, but were adjusted up by a uniform factor (1.068) to produce a total that matched the program data.

For the vaccinated population, GBS incidence rates for 7-day intervals following vaccination were calculated separately for each of the three categories of motor involvement. The cases with extensive involvement showed a sharp peak at 2 to 3 weeks after vaccination. The maximum rate was 2.47 cases per million person-weeks. By the seventh week after vaccination, the rates fell to levels consistent with estimates of a baseline incidence of GBS. This pattern was also seen when the incidence data were analyzed in terms of the timing of vaccination during the immunization program, with early, middle, and late cohorts of vaccinees compared. Incidence in the groups with either limited motor involvement or with insufficient data was consistently lower and showed no peak. The maximum weekly incidence rates in these two groups were 0.46 and 0.32, respectively.

Biweekly incidence rates for the unvaccinated population were essentially stable during the period of the immunization program, with rates for cases with extensive motor involvement consistently higher (averaging 0.14 per million person-weeks) than for those with limited involvement (averaging 0.07). These rates were adopted as "lower" estimates of baseline rates. Weekly incidence rates calculated from detailed data from Michigan and from Olmstead County, Minnesota, were adopted as "higher" estimates of baseline rates. The rate for cases with extensive motor involvement was 0.275, and the rate for cases with limited involvement was 0.13. These data were judged by the authors to reflect more complete ascertainment of cases than was achieved in the national surveillance effort.

Langmuir and colleagues calculated relative risks using both the higher and lower baseline rates for the cases with extensive motor involvement. Using the higher baseline, the relative risk for GBS during the first six 7-day intervals after receipt of the influenza vaccine was 3.96. Using the lower baseline estimate, the relative risk for that same period was 7.75. The authors reported that because they could find no basis for a more precise estimate of baseline rates, they refrained from calculating confidence intervals around these risk estimates. They calculated that the number of GBS cases attributable to the influenza vaccine was 211 with the higher baseline estimate and 246 with the lower baseline.

The authors concluded that that there was no epidemiological basis for linking the vaccinated cases with "limited" motor involvement to the swine influenza vaccine since those cases occurred without a discernable pattern. Relative risks were not calculated. Overall, limitations in the study included the inability to calculate confidence intervals because more precise baseline estimates were not found. The authors' access to only one-page summaries of the original data may have led to possible information or misclassification bias because authors were unable to verify records or check for inconsistencies or other possible mistakes.

Pennsylvania. Parkin and colleagues (1978) examined the association between swine influenza vaccination and GBS cases in Pennsylvania with onset between September 15, 1976, and January 31, 1977. The State health department identified GBS cases by contacting hospitals between December 16, 1976, and January 31, 1977, and again in March 1977 to identify late cases. In addition, mailings were sent to members of the American Boards of Psychiatry and Neurology in Pennsylvania, and news articles requested information on all cases with GBS during the onset interval of interest. For each possible case, a form was completed that included information on influenza vaccination history, date of GBS onset, lumbar puncture, mechanical respiratory assistance, death, physician contact information, and other personal information, such as race, age, and sex. Attending physicians for suspect cases were contacted and asked to provide additional information on patients meeting the case definition. GBS cases were defined as having subacute onset with full syndrome developing 1 to 7 days after initial symptoms, marked symmetrical weakness of one or both sets of extremities, and areflexia and marked hyporeflexia in areas of weakness.

Overall, about 2.9 million Pennsylvania residents (24 percent of the state's population) were vaccinated with either monovalent or bivalent influenza vaccines. The number of persons who were administered the vaccine was obtained from state and county programs as of April 1, 1977. Pennsylvania population data were based on 1970 census data.

A total of 56 cases were identified, ranging from 1 to 81 years of age, and 85 percent of these cases were evaluated by a neurologist or neurosurgeon. Two cases had GBS previously. Thirty-six cases (64%) received an influenza vaccination prior to GBS onset. Onset occurred between 1 and 102 days after vaccination, and 80 percent of vaccinated cases developed GBS within 5 weeks after vaccination. GBS was not reported in those aged 17 years or younger who were vaccinated or in those aged 65 years of older who were not vaccinated.

GBS incidence was 1.25 cases per 100,000 in the vaccinated group and was 0.22 per 100,000 in the unvaccinated group. The relative risk for the vaccinated group was 5.68. About 1 in 111,000 vaccinees developed GBS within 5 weeks after receipt of the vaccine, and about 1 in 480,000 vaccinees developed GBS more than 5 weeks after receipt of the vaccine. For the group with GBS onset within 5 weeks of influenza vaccination, the relative risk was 4.09.

About 75 percent of all cases had risk factors related to GBS, such as antecedent illness, allergies, or exposure to toxins 4 weeks prior to onset, and there was no significant difference in these factors between the vaccinated and unvaccinated groups. Severity of the syndrome and motor involvement were similar in the both groups. Three deaths occurred, all to persons who had been vaccinated. One was diagnosed with GBS 15 years earlier, and the other two had experienced an acute illness prior to onset of GBS.

The relative risks and data on timing are suggestive of an association between GBS and influenza vaccination. However, the data on other GBS risk factors did not provide clear support for a causal link with vaccination.

Ohio. Marks and Halpin (1980) examined the association between swine influenza vaccination and GBS cases in Ohio with onset between October 1, 1976, and January 31, 1977. Cases were identified by contacting all neurologists in the state who could be identified from listings of the Ohio State Medical Association or the telephone books of major metropolitan areas. Hospital-based infection control nurses were contacted by mail, with the diagnosis of any reported GBS cases verified by contacting the physician handling the case. Copies of charts or detailed summaries (information on date of onset, age, sex, extent of neurological involvement, and other clinical data) were requested for each case. GBS cases were defined as having physical evidence of bilateral, but not necessarily symmetrical, lower motor neuron weakness with an acute onset. Sensory involvement was permitted.

Overall, 2.2 million Ohio residents were vaccinated, 32 percent of the eligible population. Vaccination status of GBS cases was reported by the patient or physician. For vaccinated cases, consent forms with information on vaccine type, manufacturer, and lot number were obtained if possible. Analyses by vaccine characteristics (e.g., manufacturer or lot number) took into account total doses distributed to Ohio (about 4.9 million doses), doses administered or returned unused, and the 15 percent of distributed vaccine with unknown disposition. Ohio population data were taken from the 1970 census.

A total of 54 GBS cases were identified, all of whom had been evaluated by a neurologist. Thirty-two of the cases (58 percent) had been vaccinated, but two of them were later excluded from the analysis. The proportion of cases occurring in individuals 30 years of age or older was 96.9 percent in the vaccinated group, but only 45.5 percent in the unvaccinated group. Significantly fewer vaccinated individuals (12.9 percent) than unvaccinated cases (42.9 percent) had history of prior illness (χ^2 = 4.5; p < 0.05). There were no significant differences in other clinical characteristics. Vaccinated cases clustered in the period from late October through late December and peaked at 2 to 3 weeks after vaccination.

The incidence of GBS in the vaccinated group (13.3 per million) was significantly higher than for the unvaccinated group (2.6 per million) (χ^2 = 41.6, p = 1.6 × 10^{-10}). The relative risk for the vaccinated group was 5.1, with an attributable risk of 10.7 cases per million vaccinations. The authors also compared the rates of GBS for the vaccine from the four separate manufacturers and their individual vaccine lots. The differences among manufacturers were not significant. Using case rates calculated with person-weeks of surveillance, one vaccine lot had a significantly higher GBS rate (10 cases per 4.5 million person-weeks) than other lots (20 cases per 31.4 million person-weeks; χ^2 = 11.9, p = .0006).

The authors noted several limitations of the study in assessing causality. No standard diagnosis for GBS was available, but they found little clinical difference between cases diagnosed in vaccinated and unvaccinated persons. Case ascertainment may have been more complete in the vaccinated group, but doubling the number of cases among the unvaccinated group would still have left the rate significantly lower. With little previous epidemiologic data on GBS, it was difficult to assess the rates found in the study. The higher rate of GBS associated with a single vaccine lot might have been attributable to random variation in an analysis that included 47 different lots or to errors related to the 15 percent of vaccine without a known disposition.

Michigan. Breman and Hayner (1984) examined the incidence of GBS in Michigan between July 1, 1976, and April 30, 1977, a period that included the swine influenza vaccination program. To identify cases, neurologists, neurosurgeons, hospital record room librarians, and physical therapists were contacted via mailed questionnaire or telephone. Information on cases was also requested from primary care physicians and local health departments. Data on GBS cases were collected from December 20, 1976, to June 30, 1977. The authors noted that their methods allowed for more thorough ascertainment of GBS cases in Michigan than was achieved on the national level.

Swine influenza vaccination were based on state and national data. Overall, 2.2 million out of a population of 6.2 million persons 18 years of age and older were vaccinated in Michigan. Age- and sex-specific population estimates for the period were developed using data from the state and the U.S. Bureau of Census. Incidence rates were compared using chi-square statistics.

GBS cases were included in the study if they met the following criteria: diagnosis by a physician, bilateral muscle weakness of lower motor neuron type (with or without cranial nerve or sensory abnormalities), acute or subacute onset and evolution of signs and symptoms, and absence of other conditions (e.g., diabetes mellitus, alcoholism, and neoplasia) that could cause polyneuropathy. Patients who developed residual neurologic deficits ("chronic GBS") were included only if they met the criteria for signs and symptoms associated with onset. Information was recorded on the form developed by CDC for the national surveillance program. The patient's primary care physician or consulting neurologist was consulted to confirm the diagnosis.

A total of 300 possible cases were identified, but over half failed to meet the inclusion criteria. Vaccination status was not considered when cases were selected, but it was known to the reviewers of the records—who were epidemiologists and physicians—once review began. The review identified 132 confirmed GBS cases with onset between July 1, 1976, and June 30, 1977. The analysis was confined to 125 cases with onset before May 1, 1977, to avoid the problem of under-ascertainment of cases with onset in May and June 1977. Overall, 79 cases were unvaccinated, 8 cases had been vaccinated after the onset of GBS, 31 cases were vaccinated and had onset of GBS within 6 weeks after vaccination, and 7 cases were vaccinated and had GBS onset 7 weeks or more after vaccination. No cases occurred in vaccinated children (under 18 years of age), but 16 cases occurred in unvaccinated children.

For the vaccinated population aged 18 years or older who had onset of GBS within 6 weeks after vaccination, the incidence of GBS was 2.31 per million person-weeks, which was significantly higher than the rates in the other three groups (no p value reported). The incidence rates were 0.36 per million person-weeks in the unvaccinated group, 0.19 per million person-weeks in the group with onset before vaccination, and 0.17 per million person-weeks in the group with onset 7 weeks or more after vaccination. Using the incidence rate in the unvaccinated group as the baseline, the attributable risk for acquiring GBS within 6 weeks of vaccination was calculated to be 11.70 cases per million persons vaccinated.

In the unvaccinated group, the number of GBS cases occurring in September and October 1976 was found to be significantly greater (p <0.05) than the number of cases in the preceding and subsequent 2-month periods. The authors also compared the vaccinated and unvaccinated groups in terms of the numbers of cases occurring in November and December 1976 and the number of cases from January to April 1977. The ratio of cases in these two time periods (30 cases in November–December 1976 to 7 cases in January–April 1977) (4.3) was significantly higher than the ratio for the unvaccinated group (0.5) (p < 0.001), 9 cases in November–December 1976 to 19 cases in January–April 1977. The authors noted that this indicated that the association between vaccination and GBS onset was limited to November–December 1976 and did not extend to January–April 1977.

In other analyses, the authors found no statistically significant difference in incidence rates between the men and women, or among the vaccines from different manufacturers or with different formulations (split versus whole-cell; monovalent versus bivalent). The authors noted that the study showed an increased incidence of GBS during the swine influenza vaccination program and that the increased risk occurred for only 6 weeks after vaccination.

Michigan and Minnesota. To address persistent questions about previous analyses that had found an association between GBS and receipt of the swine influenza vaccine, Safranek and colleagues (1991) conducted a detailed review of GBS cases that occurred in Michigan and Minnesota between October 1, 1976, and January 31, 1977. About 10 percent of the 1098 cases analyzed by Schonberger and colleagues (1979) were from those two states. The analysis by Safranek and colleagues was limited to cases in persons who lived in Michigan or Minnesota and who were 18 years of age or older.

Cases were identified in two stages. First, GBS cases from Michigan and Minnesota that were reported to CDC and state health departments as part of the national surveillance effort were identified, and medical records relevant to neurological diagnosis were obtained. Second, the 424 acute care hospitals and rehabilitation facilities in the two states were asked to identify all patients discharged from October 1, 1976, through June 30, 1977, with an ICDA-8 diagnosis code 354 (a category that includes GBS). After a preliminary review, medical records were obtained for cases of possible GBS that had not been included in the original reports to CDC.

To confirm the diagnosis of GBS, the medical records for each case were reviewed by at least two neurologists from a six-member expert panel. Information on vaccination status and prior illness was masked. Diagnoses were based on standard criteria. Cases were classified as "definite," "probable," "possible," or "rejected."

Of 102 cases identified from the CDC reports, 7 were excluded from further review because the person was less than 18 years of age or because onset of GBS fell outside the reference period. The remaining 95 cases included 67 with a GBS diagnosis (48 definite, 19 probable) and 28 cases for whom the diagnosis of GBS was rejected. From the inquiries to Michigan and Minnesota hospitals and rehabilitation facilities, responses from 396 institutions (93 percent) identified

379 patients. Of these, 362 were eliminated because they did not meet clinical or nonclinical inclusion criteria. The remaining 17 were reviewed by the expert panel, and 6 were included the analysis (1 definite GBS, 2 probable, 3 possible). Thus a total of 73 cases were included in the study, of whom 67 (92 percent) had been included in the CDC analysis (Schonberger et al., 1979).

Of the 73 cases, 45 (62 percent) received the swine influenza vaccine before onset of GBS. Four cases that had been classified as unvaccinated in the CDC records were reclassified as vaccinated. Case-ascertainment in the original CDC reports was 93 percent (42/45) for vaccinated cases and 89 percent (25/28) for unvaccinated cases; the difference was not significant. For Michigan, the number of vaccinations administered each week during the immunization program was determined using estimates from the National Center for Health Statistics. For Minnesota, the numbers were based on data released as part of the 1981 court order that prompted the reanalysis of the national data (Langmuir et al., 1984). Overall, there were about 2.2 million vaccinees out of the 6.2 million adult population (36.1 percent) in Michigan. In Minnesota, there were 1.6 million vaccinees out of the population of 2.7 million (58.3 percent).

The incidence of GBS in the unvaccinated population in Michigan was 0.21 cases per million persons per week; in Minnesota, the rate was 0.38 cases per million persons per week. The difference was marginally significant ($p = 0.053$). In the vaccinated population, the rate for the 18-week surveillance period was 0.91 cases per million persons per week in Michigan and 1.10 cases per million persons per week in Minnesota. The difference was not significant ($p = 0.25$). The relative risk for GBS for the full 18-week period was 4.39 for Michigan and 2.89 for Minnesota. Looking only at the first 6 weeks following vaccination, however, the relative risk was 7.94 for Michigan and 5.23 for Minnesota (confidence intervals not reported). For the two states combined, the relative risk for 6 weeks post-vaccination was 7.10. For the vaccinated group, incidence peaked in the third week after vaccination and then declined. In contrast, the weekly incidence rate for GBS in the unvaccinated population was stable over the entire observation period. The analysis showed that Michigan had 8.6 excess GBS cases per million vaccinees attributable to vaccination and that Minnesota had 9.7 excess cases per million vaccinees.

The findings in this study were consistent with findings of earlier studies. The incidence of GBS among the vaccinated populations in Michigan and Minnesota was significantly higher than among the unvaccinated population, with a nonrandom clustering of cases in the 6 weeks following vaccination. These results were similar to the findings of Schonberger and colleagues (1979). The results of the study also showed that the CDC surveillance efforts were sensitive in detecting cases without regard to vaccination status and that over-reporting was similar both for the vaccinated and unvaccinated groups. The incidence rate seen in the unvaccinated population of these two states was similar to that in the CDC analysis. Since cases were identified if they sought medical attention or if they had a discharge diagnosis of ICD-8 354, the authors noted ascertainment bias was possible if cases in either the vaccinated or unvaccinated group were more likely to seek medical attention or to be labeled with the discharge code of ICD-8 354. Limitations in the data did not allow the authors to evaluate the extent of this bias.

Uncontrolled Observational Studies

Military Personnel. Kurland and colleagues (1986) examined data on GBS among military personnel but did not describe their methods in detail. Their analysis was based on hospitalization records of GBS cases diagnosed from 1974 to 1979 among active duty personnel serving in the U.S. Army, Navy, Marine Corps, and Air Force. Although it was not clear what sources were used to obtain the number of vaccinations administered and the number of active duty personnel serving in the military, the authors calculated that for this period an average of 80.5 percent of 2.1 million military personnel on active duty received an influenza vaccine each year. In 1976, military personnel received only whole-virus vaccine. The dose was twice the amount given to civilians.

The authors found 13 cases of GBS with onset between October 1976 and January 1977. They calculated that 30.6 cases would have been expected on the basis of the relative risk of 3.96 reported by Langmuir and colleagues (1984). The average number of cases in military personnel in any other 4-month period between 1974 and 1978 was 17.1. The average annual rate of GBS in military personnel for the 1974–1978 period was 2.4 per 100,000. No statistical analysis of the data was discussed by the authors, and the committee notes possible information bias since it was unclear what data sources were used for the number of vaccinations administered or for the number of active duty personnel serving in the military and whether these data were validated.

A previous study had examined the incidence of GBS in U.S. Army active-duty personnel, but data for 1971 through 1976 were pooled and analyzed only by month of diagnosis, not by year of diagnosis or year of vaccination. In this study, Johnson (1982) examined medical record data on GBS cases occurring in U.S. Army personnel on active duty between 1971 and 1976. Over this period, active duty Army personnel received the same or larger doses of the vaccines that were given to the civilian population. In 1976, only whole-virus influenza vaccine was used. (Active-duty Army personnel are routinely vaccinated against influenza in October, but an unknown number are missed each year. Recruits receive influenza vaccine as one of several vaccinations administered at the time they begin active duty, and thus may receive the vaccine in any month.)

Cases included in the study were admitted to the hospital between January 1, 1971, and December 31, 1976. They were identified from the Individual Patient Data System, which had records on all patients hospitalized in U.S. Army hospitals and U.S. Army personnel hospitalized at other treatment facilities. Records with several ICDA-8 diagnostic codes were requested, but all cases meeting the criteria for GBS were found to have been coded appropriately as ICDA-8 3540.

Two sets of diagnostic criteria were used. The "protocol criteria," based on those of Osler and Sidell (1960), specified symptoms of progressive motor neuropathy of unknown etiology that were severe enough to require hospitalization. Among the exclusion criteria were asymmetrical weakness, a predominance of objective sensory deficits, optic or auditory nerve involvement, or indications of active infection (fever on admission and elevated white blood count CSF). The "CDC criteria," used in the analyses of the national data (Schonberger et al., 1979; Langmuir et al., 1984), required diagnosis by a physician and objective motor deficits. No individual vaccination records were available.

A total of 127 potentially eligible hospitalization records were identified, and 114 (90 percent) were available for review. Of the records reviewed, 67 cases, including 16 recruits, fulfilled the protocol criteria for GBS. Under the CDC criteria, there were 98 cases, including 19 recruits. Depending on the diagnostic criteria used, the overall incidence of GBS ranged from about 1 to 3 cases per 100,000 per year. The number of cases was examined by month of occurrence, with data for recruits examined separately because their vaccinations were administered throughout the year. Both for recruits and non-recruits and under either set of diagnostic criteria, the greatest number of cases occurred during the first quarter of the year (January–March). The monthly pattern, however, showed no statistically significant difference from a random distribution (Edwards test for seasonality; $\chi^2 = 1.04$, $df = 2$).

The incidence of GBS in months of the first quarter of the year was 2.93 per 100,000. The rate for the months of the fourth quarter (October–December) was 1.75. On the basis of CDC's estimate of an attributable risk of 1 case per 100,000 to 120,000 vaccinees in the civilian data for October–December 1976, and assuming that up to 5,000,000 vaccinations were given to active-duty personnel, an excess of 40 to 50 GBS cases would have been expected if all Army personnel were vaccinated. Even if only 25 percent of Army personnel had been vaccinated, the author believed that any increase in GBS cases would have been evident. However, the author noted that any increased risk associated only with the 1976 vaccine in the military would have been difficult to detect. A higher underlying rate of GBS among Army personnel (based on comparisons with the rate among unvaccinated civilians) would, to some extent, mask vaccine-related risks. In addition, GBS cases that did not require hospitalization would not have been detected. Because the study examines a wide time period (1971–1976) to obtain GBS cases and does not focus solely on GBS cases occurring in 1976, the committee notes the study's limited ability in assessing GBS cases related to swine influenza vaccination.

Causality Argument

Studies that examined the association between swine influenza vaccines and GBS, including studies based on nationwide data (Schonberger et al., 1979), the reanalysis of that same data (Langmuir et al., 1984), and state-based studies (Parkin et al., 1978; Marks and Halpin, 1980; Breman and Hayner, 1984; Safranek et al., 1991) consistently showed an increased risk of GBS for the vaccinated population (See Table 3). **The committee concludes that the evidence favors acceptance of a causal relationship between 1976 swine influenza vaccines and Guillain-Barré syndrome in adults.** Concerns that the evidence of increased risk found in the original analysis of the national data might have been a reflection of inaccuracies in ascertainment of GBS cases have been addressed in subsequent studies by detailed and systematic reviews of clinical data to verify GBS diagnoses.

Although the studies of GBS among military personnel (Johnson, 1982; Kurland et al., 1986) do not show an association with the 1976 swine influenza vaccines, these studies have limitations that led the committee to discount their findings in its evaluation of the evidence. Military personnel represent a more limited age range than the civilian population and are typically healthier on average than civilians of comparable ages. In addition, information bias may have been present because estimates of the number of vaccinations administered and the number of people serving in the military were not validated and the accuracy of the data sources was not reported. Thus, these studies are limited in their ability to contribute to the causality argument.

Influenza Vaccines Used after 1976

Controlled Observational Studies

United States, 1978–1979. In 1978 a national prospective GBS surveillance system (excluding Maryland) was established by CDC, the American Academy of Neurologists (AAN), and the Conference of State and Territorial Epidemiologists. Hurwitz and colleagues (1981) used data collected through this system to examine the association between GBS and the influenza vaccine given in 1978–1979. The surveillance system was based on reports (a one-page surveillance form) submitted by neurologists to CDC on all GBS cases. Cases had to have been diagnosed by a neurologist and have objective indication of muscle involvement, with questionable diagnoses evaluated against criteria established by a committee of the NIH's National Institute of Neurologic and Communicative Disorders and Strokes.[3] The data collected on each case included demographic information, date of onset of neurologic symptoms, history of vaccination within

---

[3]The institute is now named the National Institute of Neurological Disorders and Stroke.

TABLE 3 Evidence Table: Exposure to 1976 Swine Influenza Vaccines and Guillain-Barré Syndrome

Citation	Design	Population	Assessment of Vaccine Exposure
Schonberger et al. (1979)	Cohort	U.S. population, 1976 (program targeted individuals ≥ 18 years of age, which was approximately 146 million) (based on U.S. Census Bureau data.) *Exposed:* approximately 45 million persons *GBS cases (onset 10/1/76–1/31/77):* Total = 1098 Vaccinated = 532 Unvaccinated = 558 Unknown = 8	Vaccinations per week, as reported by states to CDC NIIP Surveillance and Assessment Center. Vaccination status of GBS patients assessed by patient report; confirmation sought from copy of vaccination consent form (included type of vaccine [monovalent or bivalent] and manufacturer's lot number).

Outcomes	Results	Comment	Contribution to Causality Argument
Guillain-Barré Syndrome (GBS), with onset 10/1/76 to 1/31/77. Based on diagnosis by a physician and objective evidence of muscle involvement. Suspected cases included if accepted as a case by a state health department. Cases identified by state health department surveys of physicians, including neurologists, and hospitals. As of January 1977, CDC requested submission of standardized case information form.	*Relative Risk (95% CI) of GBS within 6 weeks after vaccination:* 0-17 years: 2.4 (0.4-16.2) 18+ years: 7.6 (6.7-8.6) All ages: 9.2 (8.2-10.3) *Attributable Risk within 6 weeks after vaccination (cases per million vaccinees):* 0-17 yrs: Not significant 18+ yrs: 8.8 All ages: 8.8 No significant differences in risk among vaccines from different manufacturers, between bivalent and monovalent vaccines, or between split- and whole-virus vaccines. Attack rate for recipients of all monovalent split-virus vaccines combined (recommended primarily for children) was significantly lower ($p < 0.5$) than the rate for recipients of all monovalent whole-virus vaccines combined. The youngest case was eleven.	Authors found (a) nonrandom distribution of intervals between vaccination and GBS onset, with cases clustered within the first 4 weeks after vaccination, and (b) lower proportion of cases with prior acute illness among the vaccinated. Clinical characteristics of the vaccinated and unvaccinated cases differed less than the attack rates in the two groups.	The study provides evidence of an association between exposure to the 1976 swine influenza vaccines and GBS in adults.

continues

TABLE 3 Continued

Citation	Design	Population	Assessment of Vaccine Exposure
Langmuir et al. (1984) Reassessment of data analyzed by Schonberger et al. (1979)	Cohort	U.S. adult population (≥ 18 years of age), 1976 *GBS cases (onset 10/1/76–1/31/77):* Total = 944 Vaccinated = 504 Unvaccinated = 440	Vaccinations per week, as reported in the National Health Survey and adjusted to match totals reported by states to CDC NIIP Surveillance and Assessment Center. Vaccination status of GBS patients as recorded in CDC records. Originally assessed by patient report; confirmation sought from copy of vaccination consent form.

Outcomes	Results	Comment	Contribution to Causality Argument
GBS, with onset 10/1/76 to 1/31/77. GBS cases categorized as having "extensive" motor involvement (n = 580); "limited" motor involvement (n= 242); or insufficient data (n=122). "Lower" estimate of baseline rates of GBS based on reported incidence in unvaccinated persons, 10/1/76-1/31/77. "Higher" estimate of baseline rates from data for Minnesota and Michigan.	*Relative Risk for GBS (extensive motor involvement) during first six 7-day intervals after receipt of the influenza vaccine:* For lower baseline estimate: 7.75 For higher baseline estimate: 3.96	Authors had access to one-page, computer-generated summaries for each of the 1098 cases in the analysis by Schonberger et al. (1979), but no access to original data. Investigators were unable to verify records or check for inconsistencies or mistakes. No confidence intervals calculated because authors could find no basis for a more precise estimate of baseline rates.	The study provides evidence of an association between exposure to the 1976 swine influenza vaccines and GBS in adults.

continues

TABLE 3 Continued

Citation	Design	Population	Assessment of Vaccine Exposure
Parkin et al. (1978)	Cohort	Pennsylvania population, based on 1970 census data. *Exposed:* 2.9 million residents (24% of state population) *GBS cases* *(onset 9/15/76–1/31/77):* Total = 56 Vaccinated = 36 Unvaccinated = 20	A short epidemiologic form including information about influenza vaccination history, was completed for each case. Attending physicians were contacted to help complete the form. Vaccines received included bivalent and monovalent products.

Outcomes	Results	Comment	Contribution to Causality Argument
GBS case defined as having subacute onset with full syndrome developing 1 to 7 days after initial symptoms, marked symmetrical weakness of one or both sets of extremities, and areflexia and marked hyporeflexia in areas of weakness. GBS cases were identified by contacting hospitals between December 16, 1976, and January 31, 1977, and again in March 1977 and identify late cases; by mailing to members of the American Boards of Psychiatry and Neurology in Pennsylvania; and by preparing news articles requesting information on all cases with GBS during the onset interval of interest.	*Relative Risk for GBS after vaccination:* 5.68 Onset within 5 weeks of influenza vaccination: 4.09 *Other related GBS risk factors:* No significant difference between vaccinated and unvaccinated.	Clustering occurred in the first 5 weeks after vaccination. About 75 percent of all cases experienced risk factors related to GBS, such as antecedent illness, allergies, or exposure to toxins 4 weeks prior to onset; there was no significant difference between the vaccinated and unvaccinated groups.	The study provides evidence of an association between exposure to the 1976 swine influenza vaccines and GBS in adults.

continues

TABLE 3 Continued

Citation	Design	Population	Assessment of Vaccine Exposure
Marks and Halpin (1980)	Cohort	Ohio population, based on 1970 census data. *Exposed:* 2.2 million residents (32% of eligible population). *GBS cases (onset 10/1/76–1/31/77):* Vaccinated = 54 (2 later excluded) Unvaccinated = 22	Vaccination status of GBS patients reported by physician or patient. Copy of consent form used as confirmation. Vaccines received included monovalent and bivalent products.

Outcomes	Results	Comment	Contribution to Causality Argument
GBS case defined as diagnosis with physical evidence of bilateral, but not necessarily symmetrical, lower-motor neuron weakness with acute onset. Sensory involvement permitted; usually mild, if present. Cellular response in CSF was usually lacking. A neurologist diagnosed all cases.	*Relative risk for GBS after vaccination:* 5.1 *Attributable risk:* 10.7 cases/million vaccinations GBS incidence in vaccinated vs. unvaccinatiod: $\chi^2 = 41.6$ p $= 1.6 \times 10^{-10}$	Possible ascertainment bias if physicians were more likely to report GBS cases in vaccine recipients than unvaccinated patients.	The study provides evidence of an association between exposure to the 1976 swine influenza vaccine and GBS in adults.

Cases were identified by contacting all neurologists listed with Ohio State Medical Association or in telephone directories for major metropolitan areas. All hospital-based infection control nurses contacted by mail, with reported cases verified by the physician.

continues

TABLE 3 Continued

Citation	Design	Population	Assessment of Vaccine Exposure
Breman and Hayner (1984)	Cohort	Michigan population, based on state and U.S. Census Bureau data.	Vaccination data based on state and national estimates.

Exposed:
2.2 million considered vaccinated (of an estimated 6.2 million persons 18 years of age or older)

*GBS cases
(onset 6/1/76-5/1/77):*
Total = 125
Unvaccinated = 79
Vaccinated:
onset before vaccination = 8
1-6 weeks after vaccination = 31
7+ weeks after vaccination = 7

Vaccination status of GBS cases determined by review of medical records by epidemiologists and physicians.

Outcomes	Results	Comment	Contribution to Causality Argument
GBS case defined as diagnosis by physician, with bilateral muscle weakness of lower motor neuron type with or without cranial nerve or sensory abnormalities; acute or subacute onset and evolution of signs and symptoms; absence of other conditions (diabetes mellitus, alcoholism, neoplasia) that could cause neuropathy. Diagnoses confirmed by primary care physician, neurologist, or both Cases identified by review of hospital discharge records for diagnosis of ICDA 354.	*GBS incidence within 6 weeks after vaccination (age 18 years or older):* Unvaccinated: 0.36 per million person-weeks Onset before vaccination: 0.19 per million person-weeks Onset 1-6 weeks after vaccination: 2.31 per million person-weeks Onset 7+ weeks after vaccination: 0.17 per million person-weeks Incidence was significantly higher in the group with onset 1-6 weeks after vaccination than in the other three groups (no p value reported). *Attributable Risk within 6 weeks after vaccination (cases per million vaccinees):* 11.70 No significant difference in incidence rates among the vaccines from different manufacturers or the different vaccine formulations.	Authors noted that the study showed an increased incidence of GBS during the swine influenza vaccination program and that the increased risk occurred for only 6 weeks after vaccination.	The study provides evidence of an association between exposure to the 1976 swine influenza vaccine and GBS in adults.

continues

TABLE 3 Continued

Citation	Design	Population	Assessment of Vaccine Exposure
Safranek et al. (1991)	Cohort	Michigan and Minnesota populations, (≥ 18 years of age), 1976. *Exposed:* Michigan: 2.2 million considered vaccinated (36.1% of total adult population). Minnesota: 1.6 million considered vaccinated (58.3% of total adult population). *GBS cases (onset 10/1/76-1/31/77):* Total: 73 Vaccinated: 45 Unvaccinated: 28	Michigan: Numbers of vaccinations administered each week during the immunization program determined from National Center for Health Statistics estimates. Minnesota: Numbers of vaccinations administered each week were based on data released under 1981 court order that prompted the reanalysis of the national data (Langmuir et al., 1984). Vaccination status of cases determined from medical records.

Outcomes	Results	Comment	Contribution to Causality Argument
GBS cases, established by expert neurology group reviewing medical records using modification of previously published criteria. Cases categorized as definite, probable, possible, or rejected. Only definites were included in the analysis. Cases identified in two stages: (1) cases from Michigan and Minnesota reported to CDC and state health departments as part of the national surveillance effort, and (2) identification by acute care hospitals and rehabilitation facilities in the two states of all patients discharged from 10/1/76 – 6/30/77 with ICDA-8 diagnosis code 354.	*Relative Risk (no CI reported):* Within 6 weeks after vaccination: Michigan: 7.94 Minnesota: 5.23 Both states: 7.10 18-week surveillance period: Michigan: 4.39 Minnesota: 2.89 For the vaccinated group, weekly incidence of GBS peaked in the 3rd week after vaccination and then declined. In the unvaccinated group, the incidence of GBS remained stable over the entire study period.	Study findings were consistent with earlier findings. Nonrandom clustering of cases in the 6 weeks following vaccination. Study also demonstrated that CDC surveillance efforts were sensitive in detecting cases without regard to vaccination status. Over-reporting similar in both the vaccinated and unvaccinated groups. Authors noted possible ascertainment bias if cases in either the vaccinated or unvaccinated group were more likely to seek medical attention or to be labeled with discharge code ICD-8 354. Limitations in the data did not allow the authors to evaluate the extent of this bias.	The study provides evidence of an association between exposure to the 1976 swine influenza vaccine and GBS in adults.

continues

TABLE 3 Continued

Citation	Design	Population	Assessment of Vaccine Exposure
Johnson (1982)	Uncontrolled observational study	U.S. military population, 1/1/1971and 12/31/1976. *Exposed* Up to 5,000,000 influenza vaccinations given to active-duty personnel. *GBS cases in U.S. Army hospital or treatment facilities between 1/1/1971-12/31/1976:* 114 records available for review.	Influenza vaccine given to all active-duty military personnel in October. Recruits immunized on entry into active duty. No individual records were available.

Outcomes	Results	Comment	Contribution to Causality Argument
Hospital records indicated ICD-8 3540 code for GBS.

Cases were further classified according to two different GBS case definitions: 1) Protocol criteria: based on Osler and Sidell (1960) diagnostic criteria that specified symptoms of progressive motor neuropathy of unknown etiology that were severe enough to require hospitalization. Exclusion criteria include asymmetrical weakness, predominance of objective sensory deficits, optic or auditory nerve involvement, or indications of active surveillance. 2) CDC Criteria: based on analyses of national data (Schonberger et al., 1979; Langmuir et al., 1984) that required diagnosis by physician and objective motor deficits. | *GBS incidence:* 1st quarter of year: 2.93/100,000

4th quarter of year: 1.75/100,000 | Any increased risk associated only with 1976 vaccine would be difficult to detect. A higher underlying rate of GBS among Army personnel would mask vaccine-related risks. In addition, GBS cases who did not require hospitalization would not have been detected. Study lacked a control group. | The study design limits the study's contribution to the causality argument. |

continues

TABLE 3 Continued

Citation	Design	Population	Assessment of Vaccine Exposure
Kurland et al. (1986)	Uncontrolled observational study	Active U.S. military personnel 1974-1978 *Exposed:* Of 2.1 million total population, 80.5 percent received vaccine each year. *GBS cases (onset 10/76-1/77):* Total: 13	Military personnel on active duty routinely receive influenza vaccine each year. No individual records available.

the 8 weeks before onset of GBS, vaccination status, date of vaccination, and type of vaccine received. The 1813 AAN neurologists participating represented 41 percent of active AAN members.

Hurwitz and colleagues (1981) studied 544 GBS cases with an onset between September 1, 1978, and March 31, 1979. Of this group, there were 12 adults ($\geq$ 18 years of age) who received the influenza vaccine within 8 weeks of the onset of GBS and 393 adults who were not vaccinated. The remaining cases, which were excluded from the analysis, included children and persons whose age or vaccination status were unknown. Of the 12 vaccinated cases, 4 (33 percent) also had an acute illness within 8 weeks of the onset of GBS. Significantly more of the unvaccinated cases, 350 of 504 patients (69 percent), had an antecedent illness (χ^2 =5.5; p < .05).

Estimates of the adult population were obtained from Census Bureau data, and estimates of the size of the vaccinated population were based on the 1979 national immunization survey. It was estimated that 8.26 percent, or 12.56 million adults, in the states covered by the surveillance system were vaccinated between September 1978 and January 1979.

Outcomes	Results	Comment	Contribution to Causality Argument
Analysis based on hospitalization records of GBS cases diagnosed 1974-1978. Average number of cases in military personnel in any other 4-month period between 1974 and 1978 was 17.1. Average annual rate of GBS in military personnel for 1974-1978 period was 2.4 per 100,000.	*GBS cases with onset between 10/76-1/77:* Expected: 30.6 Observed: 3.96	No formal statistical analysis conducted. No control group available. The committee notes possible information bias since it was unclear what the data sources were for the number of vaccinations administered or for the number of active duty personnel serving in the military and whether those data were validated.	The study's design limits the study's contribution to the causality argument.

The incidence of GBS in the vaccinated group was 0.52 cases per million persons per month, compared with 0.38 cases per million persons per month for the unvaccinated group. The relative risk of GBS for the vaccinated was 1.4 (95% CI 0.7-2.7). Allowing for the sampling error of ± 2 percent for the immunization survey, an assumption that only 6 percent of the adult population was vaccinated produces a relative risk of 1.8. The intervals from vaccination to onset were random across an 8-week period following vaccination.

The authors noted the difficulty of studying the relationship between influenza vaccine and GBS, given the rarity of GBS and the relatively small number of people who received the influenza vaccine. The detection of GBS cases was assumed to be incomplete, but the incidence rates estimated from reported cases were similar to rates from other studies. In addition, because of the well-publicized association between swine influenza vaccine and GBS, it was possible that GBS cases among persons who had been vaccinated were more likely to be reported.

United States, 1979–1980, 1980–1981. Kaplan and others (1982) used data and methods similar to those of Hurwitz and colleagues (1981) to examine the association between GBS and influenza vaccines administered in 1979–1980 and

1980–1981. Surveillance began on September 1 (before the start of the influenza vaccine campaign) and ended March 31 (8 weeks after essentially all influenza vaccine had been administered). A total of 1648 neurologists participated in 1979–1980 and 1557 neurologists participated in 1980–1981. Vaccinated GBS cases were those who had received the influenza vaccine within 8 weeks of onset of neurological symptoms. All others were considered unvaccinated.

The number of vaccinated persons was based on two sources of data. The Bureau of Census provided estimates of the adult population in the contiguous United States, minus Maryland,[4] as of June 1, 1979, and June 1, 1980. The percentage of vaccinated adults was estimated based on national immunization surveys conducted by a private research firm for the CDC. For 1979–1980, approximately 10 percent of the adult population of 153.6 million was vaccinated. For 1980–1981, approximately 9 percent of the adult population of 158.5 million was vaccinated.

For 1979–1980, a total of 528 GBS cases were reported, of which 437 were adults. Seven were vaccinated, 412 were unvaccinated, and 18 had an unknown vaccination status. For 1980–1981, a total of 459 GBS cases were reported, including 375 adult cases. Of these, 12 were vaccinated, 347 were unvaccinated, and 16 had an unknown vaccination status. The relative risk for onset of GBS within 8 weeks of vaccination was 0.6 (95% CI 0.45-1.32) in 1979–1980, and 1.4 (95% CI 0.80-1.70) in 1980–1981. The distribution of vaccinated cases by interval from vaccination to onset showed no significant clustering across the 8-week period. An analysis by age for the two seasons combined showed that the relative risk of GBS was 1.0 for vaccinated adults aged 18 to 49 years and 0.8 for adults aged 50 or older.

To assess the completeness of reporting and possible ascertainment bias, the authors investigated GBS cases that were not reported to CDC. Through telephone contacts, primarily with neurologists' office staff, an additional 354 probable cases were identified for 1980–1981. Of those cases, 4 were vaccinated within 8 weeks before GBS onset. Inclusion of these cases would have resulted in a lower estimate of the relative risk of GBS following vaccination. The committee noted that both information and ascertainment biases were possible because data for the estimated vaccinated population were not validated and estimates for the 1979-1980 population were not evaluated.

Selected States, 1992–1993, 1993–1994. Lasky and colleagues (1998) examined the association between GBS and exposure to influenza vaccines administered during 1992–1993 and 1993–1994. Data on GBS cases were obtained from hospital discharge databases from Illinois, Maryland, North Carolina, and Washington. Cases were eligible for review if onset of GBS occurred between

---

[4]Data from Maryland was not included because its GBS surveillance system is not part of the national surveillance system.

either September 1, 1992, and February 28, 1993, or September 1, 1993, and February 28, 1994. Cases classified as being definite or probable GBS were grouped and included in the analysis. Other cases were excluded. Records were reviewed by abstractors who were unaware of the case's vaccination history.

"Definite" cases had other conditions ruled out, no fever on admission (unless the fever was unrelated to GBS), symmetrical and progressive paralysis in more than one limb, areflexia or hyopreflexia in legs and arms, and an elevated CSF protein level. They either died or reached a peak of neurologic illness within 4 weeks of onset. "Probable" cases met the "definite" criteria but did not have confirming CSF data, which are not required for a GBS diagnosis. Questionable cases (e.g., those with inconsistent or missing information) were reviewed further by a neurologist. Information on patients' vaccination histories was obtained through telephone interviews with the patients or proxies. Date of vaccination was obtained from the provider. Vaccine-related GBS was defined as cases with onset of GBS within 6 weeks after receipt of the influenza vaccine.

The estimated population $\geq$ 18 years of age in the four states was 21.2 million in 1992–1993 and 21.4 million in 1993–1994. Vaccination coverage in the four states was estimated on the basis of a random-digit-dialing telephone survey. A total of 1015 adults residing in the four states responded, a response rate of about 81 percent. In 1992–1993, 4.5 million persons aged 18 years or older were vaccinated (20.9%); in 1993–1994, 5.7 million were vaccinated (26.6%) (Lasky, 2003). Response validation occurred only for positive vaccination reports from the 1993-1994 season. Validation of negative and positive vaccination reports was not conducted for the 1992-1993 season. Instead, responses were validated by comparing the change in vaccine uptake between the 1992-1993 and 1993-1994 seasons. Because Medicare reimbursements of influenza vaccine began in 1993, the change in vaccine uptake between these two seasons probably reflects increased vaccine uptake in the 65 and older age group only. GBS incidence rates were compared between the cases who were vaccinated within the 6 weeks after vaccination and the cases that occurred outside of this time period. A Poisson regression analysis was used to estimate the vaccine-related risk while controlling for age (on the basis of six age groups), vaccine season, and sex.

Out of 1201 hospital discharge records with an appropriate diagnosis code (ICD-9 357.0) for either vaccine season, 1109 were obtained for review. After exclusions for multiple admissions, residence in another state, GBS onset outside the study period, or age less than 18 years, 273 cases were available. Of this group, 180 individuals or proxies were interviewed by telephone. The rest declined to participate, could not be located, or interviews were not authorized by the patients' physicians.

A total of 19 patients were vaccinated within 6 weeks before GBS onset. There were 148 unvaccinated cases. Of these, 116 did not receive the influenza vaccine, and 32 received the vaccine outside the 6-week period preceding the onset of GBS. For six cases, permission was not given to confirm the vaccination date with a health care provider. These cases were retained in the analysis by using multiple imputation to assign a vaccination date. Seven cases whose providers could not confirm vaccination were excluded from subsequent analysis. Inclusion of two cases with plausible vaccination dates did not change the point estimate.

In the vaccinated group, GBS cases peaked during the second week following vaccination (9 of 19 cases; $p = 0.009$). Antecedent illness/infection was found less often among the vaccinated cases than the unvaccinated cases (33 percent versus 57 percent, $p = 0.06$). For the two study periods together, there were 61 million person-weeks of exposure following vaccination, and 1048 million person-weeks of non-exposure. The relative risk for GBS in vaccinated cases compared to unvaccinated cases was 2.4 (95% CI 1.5-3.8). Adjusting for sex, age group, and influenza season, the relative risk was 1.7 (95% CI 1.0-2.8). Considering the two influenza seasons separately and adjusting for sex and age group, the relative risk for GBS was 2.0 (95% CI 1.0-4.3) for 1992–1993 and 1.5 (95% CI 0.8-2.9) for 1993–1994.

The average incidence of GBS among unvaccinated adults was 0.87 case per million persons for a 6-week period. Based on the relative risk of 1.7, the estimated attributable risk in the 6-week period after vaccination was 0.61 case per million vaccinations. The authors considered this a conservative estimate, given the restrictions they imposed on including GBS cases in the analysis. After adjusting for charts not reviewed, cases excluded because of place of residence, and patients not interviewed, the attributable risk was 1.1 cases per million vaccinations. If possible cases were also included, the attributable risk would be 1.6 cases per million vaccinations.

The committee noted several study limitations. The lack of validation of vaccine status may have led to an underestimate of the number of people vaccinated in both the 1992–1993 and 1993–1994 influenza seasons. Another limitation is the loss of 13 cases due to the lack of validation of vaccination status. Recall bias of vaccine status from the 1992–1993 season is also possible since subjects were asked in 1994. Thus, although the study demonstrated a marginally significant increase in the risk of GBS after influenza vaccination, the lack of validation, the underestimation of the number vaccinated (especially in the 18-64 year age group from the 1992–1993 season), the loss of cases, and possible recall bias limit the contribution of the study to assess causality.

Military Personnel, 1980–1988. Roscelli and colleagues (1991) examined the incidence of GBS among active duty U.S. Army personnel during the period 1980–1988. GBS cases were identified from physician diagnoses in records for patients hospitalized at Army medical-treatment facilities. Army personnel are expected to receive influenza vaccine during the last week in October; the Army Surgeon General estimated a compliance rate of 80 percent for the period covered by the study.

The number of GBS cases occurring in the November months of 1980–1988 was compared with the number of cases occurring in non-November months.

Cases occurring in November were assumed to have been vaccinated and, based on previous studies, at maximum risk for vaccine-associated GBS during the 4 to 6 weeks following vaccination. For each incidence estimate, 95% confidence intervals were calculated by the normal approximation of the binomial distributions.

A total of 289 active duty Army patients were hospitalized with a diagnosis of GBS from 1980 through 1988. The mean number of cases per month in each year was 2.68. The mean number of cases for each cumulative month from 1980 to 1988 was 24.08. The total number of cases in November months was 23. In comparison, the mean number of cases in non-November months was 24.17. The authors found no significant seasonal variation.

GBS incidence rates were based a population estimate of 780,000 active duty personnel throughout the study period. In November months for 1980–1988, the incidence rate was 3.3 cases per million (95% CI 2.0-4.6). In non-November months in that same time frame, the incidence rate was 3.4 cases per million (95% CI 3.0-3.8). Based on a chi-square analysis, the difference between the two groups was not significant (p = 0.90). Making the assumption that all November cases occurred among the 80 percent of Army personnel who were assumed to be vaccinated each October, the authors estimated that the maximum vaccine-related risk for GBS was 2 cases per million vaccinations. Interpretation of the study is limited by the lack of validation of the vaccination status of GBS cases.

Unpublished Controlled Observational Studies

Selected Sites, 1990–1991. Chen (2003) presented unpublished data on the association between GBS and the influenza vaccine administered in the 1990–1991 season. Data were collected from a group of primary sites, which included Colorado, two California health maintenance organizations, and 10 sites of a Medicare demonstration program for reimbursement for influenza vaccination. The secondary sites for data collection were Louisiana and Washington. For the primary sites, cases were identified through active surveillance of practicing neurologists, plasmapheresis centers, and a review of hospital medical discharge records for diagnoses coded as ICD-9 357.0. For the secondary sites, only practicing neurologists were contacted to identify GBS cases who were included if they resided in one of the study sites at GBS onset, if onset of GBS occurred after August 1, 1990, and if age at onset was greater than 18 years. Vaccination history was obtained through an interview with the patient and validated by the patient's provider.

A total of 181 cases (9 vaccinated) were identified at the primary sites and 27 cases (3 vaccinated) at the secondary sites. Case reports were reviewed for classification as either "definite," "probable," "possible," or "rejected" on the basis of diagnostic criteria and review procedures comparable to those used by Safranek and colleagues (1991). Four neurologists served on the review panel, and two of them independently reviewed each case. Discrepancies in the classification of a case were resolved through a review and discussion by the full panel. Reports were masked for personal identifiers, vaccination status, antecedent illness, and medical epidemiologist classification.

The number of vaccine doses administered among the population aged 18 to 64 years was determined through a random digit dialing telephone survey conducted in July and August 1991. Survey participants' self-reported vaccination status was accepted without further validation. For those aged 65 years and older in the Medicare demonstration project sites, the number of vaccinations administered was determined on the basis of a separately funded vaccine coverage survey, with validation through phone, mail, or field interviews. Those results were used as a basis for extrapolating vaccination coverage in that age group in other sites. The extrapolated estimates were refined when vaccination data from the 1991 National Health Interview Survey became available. Vaccination coverage was 11 percent in the age group 18–64 years, and 48 percent in the age group 65 years or older.

For the combined population in the primary and secondary sites, the relative risk of GBS within 6 weeks of vaccination (controlled for age when appropriate) was 1.3 (95% CI 0.7-2.4). For the secondary sites alone, however, there was a significant elevation in GBS risk within 6 weeks of vaccination (RR=3.5; 95% CI 1.4-15.2). The risk of GBS within 6 weeks of vaccination was also significantly higher both in the primary and secondary sites for those aged 18 to 64 years. The overall relative risk for this age group was 3.3 (95% CI 1.7-6.5). It was 3.0 (95% CI 1.4-6.4) for the primary sites and 5.9 (95% CI 1.5-28.2) for the secondary sites. The data showed some clustering of onset within the first 4 weeks following vaccination, but there was no significant difference between the vaccinated and unvaccinated cases in antecedent illness.

Chen concluded that the data showed no increased GBS risk for the elderly (RR = 0.5, 95% CI 0.1-1.5), who were the primary target population for influenza vaccination. For the age group 18–64 years, there was an indication of increased risk for GBS following influenza vaccination, but the data on timing of GBS onset and antecedent illness did not provide clear support for a causal link with vaccination. In addition, interpretation of the study is limited by the lack of validation of vaccination status in the 18-64 year age group and the small number of cases. Overall, the committee notes that the unpublished nature of the study limits its contribution to causality.

Unpublished Uncontrolled Observational Study

Medicare Data, 1993–1994, 1994–1995. Chen (2003) also presented data from an unpublished study by Marshall McBean of the University of Minnesota School of Public Health. McBean examined the occurrence of GBS in Medicare beneficiaries (aged 65 years and older) following influenza vaccinations administered in 1993–1994 and 1994–1995. Vaccinees were identified from Medicare claims records (physician/supplier Part B bills) for influenza vaccinations administered between September 1 and December 31 of 1993 or 1994 (approximately 9.8 million in 1993 and 11 million in 1994). GBS cases were identified from hospitalization records for Medicare beneficiaries on the basis of any diagnosis coded as ICD-9-CM 357.0. Charts were abstracted according to standard protocols, and cases were classified according to criteria used by Lasky and colleagues (1998). Cases were excluded if they were hospitalized before immunization or outside the time period of interest.

For the 1993–1994 season, there was a nonrandom distribution of cases by week over a 16-week period following vaccination, with a pronounced peak during the third week. Cases following vaccinations during the 1994–1995 influenza season showed no clear pattern. Hospitalization rates for GBS during the first 6 weeks after immunization were compared with the rates for the period 7 to 16 weeks after immunization. For 1993–1994, the relative risk was 1.18 (95% CI 0.78-1.55; p = 0.59). The 1994–1995 data were not presented but were reported to show no association.

Case Reports

VAERS. Using VAERS data from 1990-1999, Geier and colleagues (2003) compared the occurrence of GBS in those who received the influenza vaccines and those who received the tetanus-diphtheria adult vaccine (Td). Numerous flaws in the study methods (unknown if vaccination status was validated, if participants received both vaccines, and if GBS was diagnosed by a neurologist) and limitations in VAERS data affect the validity and precision of the risk estimates calculated and the ability of the study's findings to contribute to causality.

At the committee's public meeting, Haber (2003) presented data on reports related to influenza vaccines that were submitted to VAERS between July 1990 and March 13, 2003. Using the indexing term "Guillain-Barré Syndrome," 565 reports of GBS were identified.[5] In a follow-up of these reports, the diagnosis of GBS was verified in 81 percent of cases, and 59 percent were reported to have occurred within 1 to 2 weeks after vaccination. Antecedent illness was reported in 18 percent of cases.

Challenge–Rechallenge Reports from VAERS. The committee reviewed four reports from VAERS that raised the possibility of the occurrence of GBS after two separate influenza vaccinations (CDC, 2003e). Reports were identified using the indexing terms "Guillain-Barré Syndrome" and "positive-rechallenge."[6] A nurse from the CDC reviewed the medical records and found that four reports were possible challenge-rechallenge cases.

---

[5]The outcome category "Guillain-Barré Syndrome" was based on indexing terms (COSTART) found in the reports, not diagnostic or medical coding terms.

[6]"Positive–rechallenge" was added as an index term in 1994.

The first case report described a 79-year-old woman who experienced "weakness, shortness of breath, and difficulty in swallowing" 3 days after influenza vaccination. The patient also experienced numbness and neuralgia, with stumbling and falling, and was admitted to the hospital. She continued to decline and was eventually diagnosed with GBS. After being released, she experienced a relapse and was readmitted to receive additional treatment. Her second admission was protracted, but she eventually recovered. The patient reported a history of GBS, with onset following a viral illness, but she reported receiving the influenza vaccine during the previous year with no subsequent adverse event.

The second report concerned a 44-year-old man with schizophrenia and a history of pneumococcal meningitis within the past 4 years. Ten days after receiving the influenza vaccine, the patient reported severe muscle pains in his shoulders and legs, followed by bilateral leg weakness and inability to stand. Clinical findings included an elevated CSF protein level and abnormal nerve conduction studies. The patient was treated with intravenous immunoglobulin. He reported that GBS had occurred after receiving influenza vaccine 12 years earlier, although no supporting information was available in the VAERS report reviewed by the committee.

A third case report was for a 44-year-old man diagnosed with GBS 37 days after receiving the influenza vaccine. The patient initially presented to the emergency room with non-radiating chest pain and numbness in the fingers and toes. After being discharged from the emergency room, the patient was later admitted with worsening weakness that progressed from the lower extremities to the trunk and upper chest, and he was diagnosed with GBS. The patient reported similar numbness in fingers and toes after first exposure to the influenza vaccine; however, no clinical documentation was available.

The fourth case report described a 33-year-old woman. Two months after receiving the influenza vaccine, the patient experienced progressive fatigue, weakness, and numbness in her extremities. Laboratory results showed normal CSF protein levels and no oligoclonal bands. Nerve conduction studies were also normal. The diagnosis recorded in the report was fibromyalgia. Three years later, the patient experienced generalized weakness and an unsteady gait about 2 months after receipt of the influenza vaccine. An MRI and EMG results were normal. The patient was again diagnosed with fibromyalgia.

The committee judged, on the basis of the supporting clinical information and the interval between receipt of the vaccine and GBS onset (3 or 10 days), that only the first two of these four reports are suggestive of cases of GBS associated with influenza vaccination. In neither of these cases, however, was the documentation sufficient to confirm GBS in response to a rechallenge with influenza vaccine.

Causality Argument

The committee reviewed several population-based surveillance studies (Hurwitz et al., 1981; Kaplan et al., 1982, Lasky et al., 1998), and a study of military personnel (Roscelli et al., 1991), and two unpublished studies that were discussed by Chen (2003) at the committee's public meeting (see Table 4). Their findings were mixed, with only one published report (Lasky et al., 1998) showing a marginally significant increase in the risk of GBS related to influenza vaccines used since 1976. The studies differed in terms of their design, the case definitions for GBS, their methods of case ascertainment, the size of the study populations, and the influenza seasons covered. Compared with the 1976 immunization experience, vaccinations were administered over a longer period of time in the years covered by these studies, making it more difficult to detect any increase that might have occurred in a rare condition like GBS. Although immunization rates were estimated to be much higher among U.S. Army personnel (Roscelli et al., 1991), the relatively small size of the population vaccinated each year would make detection of vaccine-attributable risk difficult. Because of the nature of case reports, the information from VAERS added little to the committee's ability to assess causality.

The committee concludes that the evidence is inadequate to accept or reject a causal relationship between GBS in adults and influenza vaccines administered after 1976 (that is, subsequent to the swine influenza vaccine program).

Multiple Sclerosis

The committee examined reports on epidemiological studies of the risk of MS relapses following influenza vaccination; separately it examined a smaller set of reports concerning the risk of MS onset. All these studies concerned influenza vaccines used in various years, including the swine influenza vaccines of 1976. The committee was also provided with information that 24 reports of MS[7] following influenza vaccination had been submitted to VAERS from January 1990 through March 2003 (Haber, 2003).This information did not indicate whether these reports concerned the onset of MS or relapses. As mentioned earlier, reports from passive surveillance systems like VAERS are of little assistance in assessing causality.

---

[7]The outcome category "multiple sclerosis" was based on indexing terms (COSTART) found in the reports, not diagnostic or medical coding terms.

Table 4. Evidence Table: Influenza Vaccines Used After 1976 and
Guillain-Barré Syndrome

Citation	Design	Population	Assessment of Vaccine Exposure
Hurwitz et al. (1981)	Cohort	U.S. adult population in 47 states (contiguous U.S. except MD), based on Census Bureau data as of 7/1/1978. *Exposed:* 12.56 million persons between 9/1978-1/1979 (8.26% of eligible population). *GBS cases* *(onset 9/1/1978—3/31/1979):* Total: 544 Vaccinated = 13 (12 adults) Unvaccinated = 495 (393 adults) Unknown age = 15 Unknown vaccination status = 21	Vaccinations between 8/1978 and 1/1979 estimated from 1979 national immunization survey. For GBS cases, neurologists provided vaccination history. Vaccinated cases received vaccine within 8 weeks before onset of neurological symptoms. Other cases designated as unvaccinated.
Kaplan et al. (1982)	Cohort (1979-1980)	U.S. adult population (≥ 18 years of age) in 47 states (contiguous U.S. except MD), based on Census Bureau data as of 7/1/1979 *Exposed:* 15.36 million persons (10% of eligible population) *GBS cases* *(onset 9/1/79-3/31/80):* Total: 437 Vaccinated: 7 Unvaccinated: 412 Vaccination status unknown: 18	Vaccinations between 9/1979 and 1/1980 estimated from 1980 national immunization survey. For GBS cases, neurologists provided vaccination history. Vaccinated cases received vaccine within 8 weeks before onset of neurological symptoms. Other cases designated as unvaccinated.

Outcomes	Results	Comment	Contribution to Causality Argument
GBS cases diagnosed by a neurologist with objective evidence of muscle involvement. Criteria from National Institute of Communicative Disorders and Stroke used to resolve questionable diagnoses. Cases reported to CDC by 1813 neurologists (41% of Academy of American Neurology [AAN] members).	*Relative Risk of GBS within 8 weeks of vaccination, in adults (95% CI):* 1.4 (0.7-2.7) During 8-week period before onset, antecedent illness significantly more common in the unvaccinated (69%) than in the vaccinated (33%) χ^2 =5.5; p < .05	GBS onset was random across an 8-week period following vaccination. Authors noted that the well-publicized association between swine influenza vaccine and GBS may have resulted in more complete reporting of GBS cases in the vaccinated population. Several types of vaccine were reported.	The study provides evidence of no association between exposure to influenza vaccines and GBS in adults; weaknesses in the study limit its contribution to the causality argument.
GBS cases as defined in Hurwitz et al., 1981 Cases reported to CDC as part of GBS surveillance system by 1648 neurologists who were AAN members.	*Relative Risk of GBS within 8 weeks of vaccination (95% CI):* 0.6 (0.45-1.32)	No significant clustering of cases across the 8-week period following vaccination. Similar data and methods used by Hurwitz et al. (1981) The number of vaccinated cases was based on census data and a national survey conducted by a private research firm. Possible ascertainment bias was not evaluated.	The study provides evidence of no association between exposure to the influenza vaccines and GBS in adults; weaknesses in the study limit its contribution to the causality argument.

continues

TABLE 4 Continued

Citation	Design	Population	Assessment of Vaccine Exposure
Kaplan et al. (1982) (continued)	Cohort (1980-1981)	U.S. adult population (≥ 18 years of age) in 47 states (contiguous U.S. except MD), based on Census Bureau data as of 7/1/1980.	Vaccinations between 9/1980 and 1/1981 estimated from 1981 national immunization survey.
		Exposed: 14.27 million (9% of eligible population) *GBS cases (onset 9/1/1980-3/31/1981):* Total: 375 Vaccinated: 12 Unvaccinated: 347 Vaccination status unknown: 16	For GBS cases, neurologists provided vaccination history. Vaccinated cases received vaccine within 8 weeks before onset of neurological symptoms. Other cases designated as unvaccinated.
Roscelli et al. (1991)	Cohort	Active duty U.S. Army personnel from 1980-1988 estimated to be 780,000. GBS cases with diagnosis between 1980-1988= 289 GBS cases in November months of 1980-1988 compared to non-November months.	Vaccination information from office of the Surgeon General of the US Army. About 80%of all active duty soldiers were vaccinated in the last week of October from 1980-1988.

Outcomes	Results	Comment	Contribution to Causality Argument
GBS cases as defined in Hurwitz et al., 1981 Cases reported to CDC as part of GBS surveillance system by 1557 neurologists who were AAN members.	*Relative Risk of GBS within 8 weeks of vaccination (95% CI):* 1.4 (0.80-1.76) *Relative Risk of GBS within 8 weeks of vaccination by age group (95% CI) 1979-1980 and 1980-1981 data combined:* 18-49 years: 1.0 50 years or older: 0.8	No significant clustering of cases across the 8-week period following vaccination. Similar data and methods used by Hurwitz et al. (1981) The number of vaccinated cases was based on census data and a national survey conducted by a private research firm. Evidence of some underreporting of unvaccinated cases suggested possible overestimate of risk of GBS for vaccinated population.	The study provides evidence of no association between exposure to influenza vaccines and GBS in adults; weaknesses in the study limit its contribution to the causality argument.
GBS cases hospitalized at Army Medical Treatment Facilities between 1980-1988. Cases identified from physician diagnoses in medical records.	*GBS Incidence per 10^6* Novembers, 1980-1988: 3.3 (95% CI 2.0-4.6) Non-November months, 1980-1988: 3.4 (95% CI 3.0-3.8) Chi-square: difference was not significant (p=0.90)	Interpretation of the study is limited by lack of validation of the vaccination status of GBS cases.	The study design limits the study's contribution to the causality argument.

continues

TABLE 4 Continued

Citation	Design	Population	Assessment of Vaccine Exposure
Lasky et al. (1998)	Cohort	Adult population in Illinois, Maryland, North Carolina, and Washington, 1992 and 1993. *Exposed:* 1992-1993: 4.5 million 1993-1994: 5.7 million *Definite or probable GBS (onset between 9/1/1992 and 2/28/1993 or between 9/1/1993 and 2/28/1994):* Total = 180 Vaccinated = 19 Not vaccinated = 148 Vaccination status unconfirmed = 13	Vaccination coverage in the 4 states was estimated on the basis of a random-digit-dialing telephone survey. Vaccination history of GBS patients determined through telephone interviews with patients or proxies. Providers contacted to obtain exact dates of vaccination. Vaccine-associated cases defined a priori as those with onset of GBS within 6-week period after vaccination.

Outcomes	Results	Comment	Contribution to Causality Argument
GBS cases identified from hospital discharge database records with ICD-9 diagnosis 357.0. Cases were categorized as definite, probable, or possible GBS, not GBS, or requiring review. Identification of definite and probable cases based on published diagnostic criteria. Only definite and probable cases included in the analysis.	*Relative Risk of GBS within 6-weeks after influenza vaccination (95% CI):* 2.4 (1.5-3.8) Adjustment for age, sex, and season: 1.7 (1.0-2.8) Relative Risk (95%CI) controlling for age and sex 1992-1993: 2.0 (1.0-4.3) 1993-1994: 1.5 (0.8-2.9)	Of 1201 records reviewed, most were excluded because of multiple admissions, residence in another state, GBS onset outside study period, age less than 18 years, declined to participate, could not be located, or interview not authorized by patient's physician. Committee notes that loss of 13 cases because of lack of validation of vaccination status limits the strength of the study's findings. In addition the lack of validation of vaccine status may have led to an underestimate of the number of people vaccinated in both the 1992-1993 and 1993-1994 influenza seasons. Recall bias of vaccine status from the 1992-1993 season is also possible since subjects were asked in 1994.	The study provides evidence of a marginally significant association; weaknesses in the study limit its contribution to the causality argument.

continues

TABLE 4 Continued

Citation	Design	Population	Assessment of Vaccine Exposure
Chen, 2003 (Unpublished)	Cohort	Adult population (≥18 years) in primary study sites (CO, 2 CA HMOs, 10 Medicare demonstration sites) and secondary sites (LA, WA), 1990-1991 influenza season. GBS cases with onset after 8/1/1990. Age at onset greater than 18 years of age. *GBS cases at primary sites:* Total = 181 Vaccinated = 9 *GBS cases at secondary sites=* Total = 27 Vaccinated = 3	Number of vaccine doses administered in population aged 18-64 years determined through random digit telephone survey. Self-reported vaccination status without validation was accepted. For persons aged 65 years and older at Medicare demonstration project sites, the number of vaccinations administered was determined on the basis of vaccine coverage survey, which was validated. Vaccination data also available from NHIS. Vaccination coverage: 18-64 years: 11% 65 years or older: 48%
McBean, 2003 (Unpublished) Presented by Chen (2003) to Immunization Safety Review Committee	Uncontrolled observational	Medicare beneficiaries (aged 65 years and older), 1993-1995 Total influenza vaccine recipients: 9.8 million *Number of GBS cases hospitalized* *Within 6 weeks of vaccination = 19* *Between 7-16 weeks after vaccination = 26*	Vaccinees identified from Medicare claims records (physician/supplier Part B bills) for influenza vaccinations administered 9/1/1993-12/31/1993 and 9/1/1994-12/31/1994.

Outcomes	Results	Comment	Contribution to Causality Argument
GBS cases identified using criteria of Safranek et al. (1991). Neurologists reviewed each case, which were classified as either definite, probable, possible, or rejected. Cases from primary sites were identified through active surveillance of practicing neurologists, plasmapherisis centers, and hospital discharge records with diagnosis code of ICD-9 357.0. For secondary sites, only practicing neurologists were contacted.	*Relative risk of GBS within 6 weeks of influenza vaccination (95%CI)* Both primary and secondary sites: > 18 years: 1.3 (0.7-2.4) 18-64 years: 3.3 (1.7-6.5) > 65 years: 0.6 (0.1-1.5) Primary sites alone: > 18 years: 1.1 (0.5-2.1) 18-64 years: 3.0 (1.4-6.4) > 65 years: 0.3 (0.1-1.3) Secondary sites alone: > 18 years: 3.5 (1.4-15.2) 18-64 years: 5.9 (1.5-28.2) > 65 years: 1.8 (0.2-14.7) Some clustering of onset within the first 4 weeks following vaccination No significant difference between vaccinated and unvaccinated cases in antecedent illness.	Interpretation of the study's findings are limited by the lack of validation of vaccination status in the 18-64 age group. Data on timing and antecedent illness did not provide clear support for a causal link.	The study suggests an association between exposure to influenza vaccines and GBS in adults; as an unpublished study, its contribution to the causality argument is limited.
GBS cases identified from hospitalization records for Medicare beneficiaries on basis of any diagnosis coded as ICD-9-CM 357.0. Cases were classified according to criteria used by Lasky et al. (1998)	*Relative risk of hospitalization for GBS during the first 6 weeks after immunization vs. 7-16 weeks after immunization (95%CI):* 1993-1994: 1.7 (0.78-1.55, p=0.59) 1994-1995: data not presented, but reported to show no association.	No control group.	The study design and its unpublished status limit its contribution to the causality argument.

continues

TABLE 4 Continued

Citation	Design	Population	Assessment of Vaccine Exposure
Geier et al., (2003)	Cohort	Cases: GBS after influenza vaccination "Controls": GBS after Td (adult) vaccination. Number not reported.	Based on VAERS data. Biological Surveillance Summary data provided the number of influenza vaccine doses administered (distributed?) by manufacturer and year.
CDC (2003e)	Case series	Case reports submitted to VAERS between July 1990 and March 2003.	Receipt of influenza vaccine as reported to VAERS.

Outcomes	Results	Comment	Contribution to Causality Argument
Severe GBS defined as a case of GBS with only partial recovery and significant residual disability 1 year later.	*Relative risk (95%CI) of GBS after influenza immunization compared to GBS after Td immunization by year:* 1992 4.9 (1.2-20.2) 1993 12.5 (3.0-50.4) 1994 6.4 (1.6-27.0) 1995 4.8 (1.7-12.9) 1996 3.3 (1.5-7.2) 1997 3.4 (1.1-11.4) 1998 2.0 (0.84-4.7) 1999 4.2 (0.81-14.3) *Attributable Risk by year* 1992 3.9 1993 11.5 1994 5.4 1995 3.8 1996 2.3 1997 2.4 1998 1.0 1999 3.2	The committee notes that it is unknown if vaccination was validated, if GBS was diagnosed by neurologist, and if participants received both vaccines. Limitations in VAERS data affect the validity and precision of the risk estimates calculated.	The study design and limitations of VAERS data restrict the study's contribution to the causality argument.
Reports were included when the indexing term "Guillain-Barré syndrome" was noted in the VAERS report. Cases identified on the basis of inclusion of GBS as indexing term.	*Number of GBS reports* 565 Diagnosis verified: 81% Occurrence within 1-2 weeks after vaccination: 59% Antecedent illness reported: 18%	The analytical value of data from passive surveillance systems is limited by such problems as underreporting, lack of detail, inconsistent diagnostic criteria, and inadequate denominator data (Ellenberg and Chen, 1997; Singleton et al., 1999).	The nature of VAERS reports limits their contribution to the causality argument.

continues

TABLE 4 Continued

Citation	Design	Population	Assessment of Vaccine Exposure
VAERS: Possible challenge-rechallenge	Case-reports	Case reports submitted to VAERS, July 1990-March 2003. Four reports of GBS identified as possible rechallange.	Receipt of influenza vaccine listed in record.as reported in VAERS

Outcomes	Results	Comment	Contribution to Causality Argument
GBS following influenza vaccination with history of GBS. Cases identified on the basis of inclusion of "GBS" and "positive rechallenge" as indexing terms and review of records by CDC nurse.	Case #1: 79-year-old experienced "weakness, shortness of breath, and difficulty in swallowing" 3 days after influenza vaccination. Patient reported history of GBS, with onset following viral illness. Reported influenza vaccination during the previous year with no subsequent adverse events. Case #2: 44-year-old man with schizophrenia and history of pneumococcal meningitis. Ten days after receiving influenza vaccine reported severe muscle pains in his limbs followed by bilateral weakness in his legs and inability to stand. He reported GBS after receiving influenza vaccine 12 years earlier, but no supporting information was available in the VAERS report reviewed by the committee. Case #3: 44-year-old man diagnosed with GBS 37 days after influenza vaccination. The patient presented with non-radiating chest pain and numbness in fingers and toes. Patient was later admitted with worsening weakness. Reported similar numbness in fingers and toes after first influenza vaccine exposure; however, no clinical documentation was available.	The committee judged, on the basis of the supporting clinical information and the interval between vaccination and GBS onset (3 or 10 days), that only cases 1 and 2 are suggestive of GBS associated with influenza vaccination. In neither of these cases, however, was the documentation sufficient to confirm GBS in response to a rechallenge with influenza vaccine.	The nature of VAERS reports limits their contribution to the causality argument.

continues

TABLE 4 Continued

Citation	Design	Population	Assessment of Vaccine Exposure
VAERS: Possible challenge-rechallenge (continued)			

MS Relapse: Randomized Controlled Trials

California, 1976. Myers and colleagues (1977) conducted a randomized controlled trial to examine the safety and efficacy of the 1976 swine influenza vaccine in MS patients. Subjects were recruited from two MS clinics in the Los Angeles area and the private practice of a Los Angeles neurologist. Excluded from the study were patients who were under 24 years of age, were receiving immunomodulating medications, or had a history of an allergic reaction to eggs or previous influenza vaccinations. The age range of subjects was 26-64 years. An initial pilot study with 10 influenza-vaccinated patients and 10 placebo-inoculated patients found no differences in local and systemic reactions between the two groups.

The second phase involved three groups: vaccine recipients (n = 23), placebo recipients (n = 23), and untreated controls (n = 22). Assignment to a group was based on restrictive randomization. Patients were first classified as having active or inactive MS. Active MS was defined as a relapse in the preceding 3 months or deterioration over the past 6 months. All other patients were defined as having inactive MS. Patients in each group were then randomly assigned to receive either the swine influenza vaccine (a bivalent, whole-virus product) or the placebo (vaccine diluent without virus). Before the injections were given, each patient was evaluated by a neurologist to document the course and phase of the person's disease and assign a functional systems and disability status score.

Outcomes	Results	Comment	Contribution to Causality Argument
	Case #4: 33-year-old woman experienced progressive fatigue, weakness, and numbness in extremities 2 months after influenza vaccination. Diagnosis reported was fibromyalgia. Three years later the patient experienced weakness and unsteady gait about 2 months after influenza vaccination. MRI and EMG results were normal, and the patient was diagnosed with fibromyalgia.		

Vaccination status was unknown both to patients and researchers. Adverse events were identified by patient reports and evaluations by a neurologist at 3 weeks and 3 months after injection. Local and systemic reactions were reported by 52 percent of vaccine recipients, compared with 25 percent of placebo recipients. One vaccinated patient developed a mild, immediate hypersensitivity reaction, with localized pain and a local area of erythema.

In each of the three study groups, four patients experienced relapses within the 3 months following injection. For three patients each in the vaccine and placebo groups and one patient in the untreated group, relapse involved myelopathy with weakness, sensory loss, and ataxia in lower extremities. Among the vaccine recipients, three of the relapses were mild and one was moderate. Among the placebo recipients, two experienced a moderate relapse and one experienced a severe relapse. All of the relapses were mild among the control group.

The relapse rate was 0.5 case per patient per year for the vaccine recipients and 0.7 case per patient per year for the placebo group. Based on the similar relapse rates among the groups, the authors concluded that exposure to the influenza vaccine was safe for MS patients.

Northeastern MS Centers, 1993. Miller and colleagues (1997) conducted a multicenter, randomized controlled trial to examine the association between receipt of influenza vaccine and exacerbation of relapsing-remitting MS. The study was conducted during the influenza season of 1993.

Subjects were recruited from five MS centers in northeastern states. Patients were eligible for the study if they had a clinically definite case of relapsing-remitting multiple sclerosis with a Kurtzke expanded disability status score (EDSS) of less than 6.5 (able to walk with minimal assistance). Patients were excluded if they had acute exacerbations or treatment with corticosteroids in the previous 4 weeks; treatment with immunosuppressive medications, interferon-beta, or copolymer 1 within the preceding 6 months; or a history of prior adverse reactions to influenza vaccine or an allergy to egg products.

A total of 104 patients were randomized to receive either standard influenza vaccine from a single manufacturer or a placebo. Each of the five centers had its own randomization sequence. Both investigators and subjects were blinded to vaccination status. Participants were followed for 6 months, with examinations by a neurologist at 4 weeks and at 6 months after inoculation. An MS exacerbation was defined as a demonstrated change observed during a neurologic examination, measured as an increase of at least 0.5 on the EDSS, at least one grade on the scores of two or more of the Kurtzke functional system scores, or two grades on one of the functional system scores. Neurologic changes had to persist for more than 24 hours (or more than 48 hours after a fever). Sample size was calculated for detection of a moderate effect size, assuming an alpha of 0.05 with a 2-tailed test and a power of 80 percent.

Forty-nine participants received the influenza vaccine, and 54 received the placebo injection. The groups were similar in age (ages of subjects were not reported), gender, and disability. After 28 days, three vaccine recipients and two placebo recipients had experienced exacerbations, a difference that the authors reported was not significant (Fisher's exact test). After 6 months, vaccine recipients had experienced 11 exacerbations (an annual rate of 0.45) compared with 6 among the placebo recipients (annual rate 0.22). The difference was not significant (chi-square analysis). The mean change in disability status score (vaccine = 0.02, placebo = 0.09) was not significantly different between the two groups (based on t-test for independent samples). The authors concluded that the vaccine did not appear to be associated with an increased risk of MS relapse.

MS Relapse: Controlled Observational Studies

Arizona, 1976. Bamford and colleagues (1978) examined the effect of the 1976 swine influenza vaccine on MS patients receiving care at the MS clinic of the Arizona Health Sciences Center. These patients were examined on a regular basis at the clinic, and their disability rated with the Kurtzke Disability Status Scale. A bivalent swine influenza vaccine was used in the study.

A total of 127 patients were assessed during November and December 1976 (ages of subjects were not reported). Of this group, 65 patients elected to receive the vaccine, and 62 served as unvaccinated controls. The two groups were described as similar in terms of levels of disability and disease course. Patients were interviewed during the month following vaccination and asked about any new neurologic symptoms, deterioration of existing symptoms, or (among vaccinated patients) any allergic or toxic reactions to the vaccine. Two patients reported systemic symptoms following vaccination. The vaccinated group also had one patient with onset of a new neurologic symptom and one patient with increased severity of an existing dysfunction. In the unvaccinated group, two patients had new symptoms and two had increased disability.

The vaccine recipients experienced 0.031 episodes of deterioration per patient-month of exposure, compared with 0.032 episodes per patient-month for the unvaccinated group. No statistical tests were reported. The authors noted that the occurrence of symptoms was similar to findings from other studies and concluded that the vaccine did not seem to affect individuals already diagnosed with MS. Other study limitations include the short time frame (four weeks) between vaccination and reporting of outcome, and patients self-selecting to receive the vaccine and self-reporting outcomes.

New York, 1993. Mokhtarian and colleagues (1997) examined the safety and efficacy of influenza vaccination for MS patients in a double-blind clinical trial sponsored by the MS Society. Eligible patients had a diagnosis of clinically definite relapsing-remitting MS and a Kurtzke Extended Disability Status Score (EDSS) of less than 6.5. Exclusion was based on a Kurtzke score of ≥ 6.5, an acute exacerbation within the previous 4 weeks, treatment with immunosuppressive medications within the previous 6 months, or a history of allergy to influenza vaccine or eggs. A single neurologist examined all participants before and after inoculation. Patients were evaluated at 4 weeks and followed for 6 months. They were asked to report any clinical exacerbations or the occurrence of influenza.

The study participants included 19 MS patients, ranging in age from 28 to 60 years, and 9 age- and sex-matched subjects without MS. Trivalent influenza vaccine prepared by a single manufacturer for the 1993–1994 season was given to 11 MS patients and the 9 participants without MS. The remaining 8 MS patients received a placebo (vaccine diluent). No randomization procedures were reported.

Overall, three exacerbations occurred among influenza-vaccinated MS patients, at 19, 98, and 177 days after vaccination. The authors noted that the two late-occurring exacerbations may not have been related to the vaccination. In the placebo group, two MS patients experienced attacks at 22 and 43 days after inoculation. Overall, there was no significant difference in EDSS at the beginning and the end of the study for either the placebo- or influenza-vaccinated groups. Flu-like symptoms were reported by two influenza-vaccinated MS patients (44 and 90 days after vaccination), one placebo-vaccinated MS patient, and one influenza-vaccinated subject without MS (20 days post-vaccination).

The authors concluded that the study provided no indication that influenza vaccine was associated with exacerbation of MS in patients with an EDSS of less than 6.5, but the effectiveness of the vaccine in preventing influenza illness was unclear. The authors note limitations related to the small size of the study population. Interpretation of the results is also hindered by the lack of formal statistical analysis of differences between the vaccine and placebo groups.

Vaccines in Multiple Sclerosis (VACCIMUS)—France, Spain, and Switzerland. Confavreux and others (2001) conducted a multicenter case-crossover study to examine whether vaccination increases the risk of relapse in MS. The study subjects were MS patients from neurology departments associated with the European Database for Multiple Sclerosis network. With the case-crossover design, patients served as their own controls. Those eligible for the study had a definite or probable diagnosis of MS according to the Poser criteria (Poser et al., 1983) and had at least one relapse between January 1993 and December 1997. The index relapse was the first during this period that was confirmed by a medical visit or hospitalization and that was preceded by a relapse-free period of 12 months. Neurologists reviewed patients' medical records to confirm the diagnosis of MS and categorized the index relapse as either definite, probable, or possible. A total of 643 subjects were included in the study.

Vaccination histories during the period January 1992 through December 1997 were collected from study subjects by telephone interview and confirmed with written documentation, usually a copy of the vaccination record. Vaccine exposures included influenza, hepatitis B, tetanus, hepatitis A, typhoid, yellow fever, typhoid-paratyphoid, tetanus-poliovirus, tetanus-diphtheria, and tetanus-poliovirus-diphtheria vaccines. During the 12 months before the index relapse, 135 subjects had a confirmed vaccination of any sort, and 23 had a confirmed influenza vaccination. Influenza vaccination exposure was assessed in terms of a 2-month risk period immediately before the index relapse and four 2-month control periods during the 10 months preceding the index relapse.

A conditional regression analysis was used to calculate the relative risk of MS relapse associated with exposure to the influenza vaccine or to other vaccines. For influenza vaccination, the relative risk of relapse was 1.08 (95% CI, 0.37–3.10); the relative risk of relapse associated with any vaccine exposure was 0.71 (95% CI, 0.40–1.26). The authors concluded that vaccination does not increase the short-term risk of a relapse among patients with MS who had been relapse-free for at least 12 months. However, the authors noted that the study findings are inconclusive with regard to long-term risks.

Limitations cited by the authors include lower power for assessing risks associated with specific vaccines, exclusion of those patients with frequent or minor relapses, and an assumption of constancy of vaccine exposure and equality of risk after each exposure. Study strengths included limited confounding by the nature of the case-crossover study design, high response rates and validation of vaccine exposures, limited recall bias through collection of exposure data without specific reference to the index relapse, and results that are unaffected by a change in length of effect periods.

The committee notes that the relative risk of 1.08 may reflect not only the effect of the influenza vaccine on MS relapse, but also the adverse effect of acute illnesses. Unlike other vaccines, which are administered throughout the year, influenza vaccine is generally given only during autumn and winter, a time when acute illnesses are also more prevalent. Thus, during the risk period of interest, MS patients may be receiving the influenza vaccine and experiencing respiratory illness. The relative risk reported by the study may be an overestimate of the risk of MS relapse associated with influenza vaccine, as it is based on a risk interval when both influenza vaccination and acute illnesses may occur.

Kurland and others (1984) report unpublished data by Brooks and colleagues (unpublished, 1980) of MS relapse between 31 MS patients and 28 controls without MS, matched according to sex and age. Frequency of exacerbations was compared 3 months before and 21 months after receipt of the influenza vaccination. There was no increase in exacerbation rate either before or after vaccination.

MS Relapse: Uncontrolled Observational Studies

Arizona. Sibley and colleagues (1976) examined the effect of polyvalent influenza vaccinations received between 1962 and 1975 on MS patients treated at the Multiple Sclerosis Clinic at the University of Arizona Medical Center. Records of 128 current patients were reviewed for history of influenza vaccination and subsequent deterioration of MS symptoms. Patients were also interviewed about reactions to vaccination, such as fever, allergic reactions, headaches, and symptoms that suggested an attack of MS. Neurological symptoms occurring within the month after vaccination were considered vaccine-related. Also included in the study were data on 24 other MS patients who had received a polyvalent influenza vaccine in 1962.

Of the 152 patients in the study (ages of subjects were not reported), 93 patients had received 209 influenza vaccinations at various times between 1962 and 1975. Vaccine-related reactions occurred among 19 percent of patients. The authors noted that the observed rate of relapse (1 attack in 93 patient-months of observation) was less than expected for the natural course of the disease (4.5 exacerbations per month). Limitations in the study include the lack of a comparison control group. In addition, no formal statistical analysis was conducted.

The Netherlands, 1996. De Keyser and colleagues (1998) compared the effects of influenza vaccine and the effects of influenza illness on patients with either primary progressive MS or relapsing MS. Primary progressive MS was defined as a progressive course from onset, without superimposed exacerbations. The category of relapsing MS included the relapsing-remitting form, with or without secondary progression, and the progressive-relapsing form.

In December 1996, questionnaires were sent to 320 MS patients listed in the Groningen MS Databank. Information was collected on age, sex, form of MS, severity of disability, and duration of the disease. Patients were asked if they had experienced influenza illness between November 1995 and February 1996 or received influenza vaccine in autumn of 1996 (the trivalent product for the 1996–

1997 influenza season). They were also asked if they had experienced any worsening or exacerbation of their MS in the 6 weeks following either influenza illness or vaccination. Differences in relapse rates were compared using Fisher's exact test.

Responses were received from 233 patients (74 percent), including 53 with primary progressive MS and 180 with relapsing MS. The mean age of subjects was 44 years. In the primary progressive group, 4 patients had experienced influenza illness and 24 had been vaccinated. None of the vaccinated patients reported an effect on neurologic symptoms. Among the 180 relapsing MS patients, 36 had experienced influenza illness and 70 had been vaccinated. Twelve patients (33 percent) reported exacerbations after influenza illness, whereas only 4 patients (5 percent) experienced exacerbations in the 6 weeks after vaccination ($p < 0.0001$). For the 48 relapsing MS patients restricted to wheelchair use (those with greater disability), the incidence exacerbation following vaccination (1 of 42 patients) was also significantly lower than that following illness (3 of 4 patients) ($p = 0.001$). The authors noted that the post-immunization relapse rate was similar to that found in other studies. They acknowledged that some patients reporting illness may have had a disease other than influenza.

MS Relapse: Case Series

Italy. Salvetti and colleagues (1995) evaluated a series of six patients with clinically definite MS who received influenza vaccine (age range of subjects was between 25-40 years of age). Patients were clinically evaluated every 3 months during the year preceding vaccination with trivalent inactivated influenza vaccine and the year following receipt. Gadolinium-enhanced magnetic resonance imaging (GD-MRI) was performed 1 day before vaccination and 15 and 45 days after vaccination to assess whether changes in the permeability of the blood–brain barrier were evident following vaccination.

Five patients experienced the same or a lower number of relapses following vaccination than during the preceding year. These patients also showed no increase in the progression of disability, based on the EDSS. One patient experienced a shift from the relapsing-remitting form of MS to the progressive form during the year after vaccination. This patient was also the only one with new lesion evident on the GD-MRI (at 15 days post-vaccination). The other patients had unremarkable GD-MRI scans after vaccination. As a case-series report, this study makes a limited contribution to the causality assessment.

Incident MS: Controlled Observational Study

United States—Vaccine Safety Datalink. DeStefano and colleagues (2003) conducted a case-control study to examine the relationship in adults between vaccination and the development of MS and optic neuritis; the study also examined the risk related to the timing of vaccination. The results for MS are discussed here and those for optic neuritis are discussed below. Data for both cases and controls were obtained from three health maintenance organizations (HMOs) that participate in CDC's Vaccine Safety Datalink (VSD) project. Automated outpatient and hospital discharge data for 1995–1999 were screened, and cases were confirmed by review of medical records. Cases were defined as having any physician's diagnosis of MS or optic neuritis on their medical records. Alternative definitions were a diagnosis by a specialist or the meeting of the International Panel criteria for MS (two demyelinating episodes separated in space and time). Up to three controls were selected for each case and matched according to year of HMO enrollment (minimum membership of 1 year), age, and sex. Patients who had a prior diagnosis of MS or optic neuritis in their medical charts were excluded. A total of 440 cases (332 with MS and 108 with optic neuritis) and 950 controls (722 controls for MS cases and 228 controls for ON cases) participated in the study.

Influenza vaccine exposure was determined on the basis of medical chart reviews and telephone interviews (for those vaccinated outside the HMO). Exposure was categorized as ever or never vaccinated before the index date (i.e., the date of onset for the matched case). The time intervals between vaccination and the index date were 0–1 year, 1–5 years, and more than 5 years. Of the cases, 16.6 percent had received a influenza vaccination before the index date; of the controls, 18.6 percent had been vaccinated.

Odds ratios were calculated using a conditional logistic regression stratified by matching variables and adjusted for family history, race and ethnicity, place of birth, Scandinavian ancestry, smoking, and marital status. Using the case definition based on the presence in the medical record of a physician's diagnosis of MS, the risk of MS following influenza vaccination was OR = 0.7 (95% CI, 0.5-1.1). Similar results were obtained using case definitions based on specialist diagnosis: for MS and optic neuritis combined, the odds ratio was 0.9 (95% CI, 0.6-1.3). With the International Panel criteria for diagnosis of MS the odds ratio was 1.0 (95% CI, 0.6-1.4). The adjusted odds ratios for timing of influenza vaccination and risk of demyelinating disease (MS and optic neuritis combined) was 0.8 (95% CI, 0.5-1.4) for less than 1 year before index date, 1.1 (95% CI, 0.7-1.7) for 1 to 5 years before the index date, and 0.6 (95% CI, 0.3-1.1) for more than 5 years before the index date.

The authors concluded that the results did not support the hypothesis that influenza vaccination causes or triggers the development of MS. The authors cited as strengths of the study identifying cases and controls from the large HMO population covered by the VSD project, minimizing recall bias by focusing on recently diagnosed cases, using medical records to establish the timing of onset of MS and of vaccination, and having obtained consistent results with different case definitions. A limitation of the study was the need to rely on self-report to obtain information on vaccinations obtained outside the HMOs. About half of both cases and controls received such vaccinations, but excluding the self-reported data had little effect on the results.

Incident MS: Uncontrolled Observational Study

U.S. Army. Kurland and colleagues (1984) reviewed data on new cases of MS diagnosed among U.S. Army personnel from 1975 through 1979. The number of new cases occurring following administration of the swine influenza vaccine in autumn of 1976 was compared with the number occurring at other times during the 1975–1979 period. Influenza vaccinations are administered to active duty personnel each year in October and are administered to new recruits throughout the year when they begin service. Between 765,000 and 779,000 persons were on active duty in these years, and an estimated 85 percent received the swine influenza vaccine in 1976. The average number of new MS cases per calendar quarter was 6.55. Five cases were diagnosed during the final quarter of 1976 and 6 during the first quarter of 1977. During the seven calendar quarters preceding the 1976 influenza vaccinations, 57 cases of MS were diagnosed; during the final quarter of 1976 and the next six quarters, 45 cases were diagnosed. The authors interpret these data as indicating that the 1976 influenza vaccine did not affect the immediate or longer-term risk of developing MS among U.S. Army personnel.

Causality Argument

On the basis of the Confavreaux study (2001) and the consistent findings from the other studies (Miller et al., 1997; Mokhtarian et al., 1997; Bamford et al., 1978; Myers et al., 1977) (see Table 5), **the committee concludes that the evidence favors rejection of a causal relationship between influenza vaccines and relapse of multiple sclerosis in adults.** Uncontrolled studies and case series (De Keyser, 1998; Salvetti et al., 1995; Sibley et al., 1976) provide similar findings, but given their nature they are of limited value in assessing causality. The occurrence of relapse is rare and the power to detect increased risk is limited.

Few studies have examined the association between influenza vaccination and the onset of MS. Only one study (DeStefano et al., 2003) provided a thorough description of the study methods and outcomes (see Table 6). It found no increase in the risk of onset of MS associated with influenza vaccination, but in the absence of confirmation from other sources, **the committee concludes that the evidence is inadequate to accept or reject a causal relationship between influenza vaccines and incident MS in adults.** However, the biological mechanisms involved in the onset of MS are presumed to be related to those involved in relapse. With the epidemiological data favoring the rejection of a causal relationship between influenza vaccines and relapse of MS, the committee sees no reason to suspect that a causal relationship might exist between influenza vaccines and onset of MS.

Because the available studies did not consistently report ages (some did not report age at all, and detail is lacking in studies that did report age, for example, reporting average age without a range) and none of the studies specifically included children, the committee could not reach a conclusion on causality in the children's age group, but also could not clearly define the lower age limit for its conclusion in adults.

Optic Neuritis

Controlled Observational Study

United States—Vaccine Safety Datalink. As described above, DeStefano and colleagues (2003) conducted a case-control study examining the relationship in adults between influenza vaccination and the development of the central nervous system demyelinating diseases MS and optic neuritis. The study also examined the risk related to the timing of vaccination. The results for optic neuritis are discussed here; the results for MS are discussed above.

Automated HMO outpatient and hospital discharge data for 1995–1999 were screened to select cases and controls, and cases were confirmed by review of medical records. For optic neuritis, cases were defined as having any physician's diagnosis of optic neuritis in their medical records, or alternatively a diagnosis by a specialist. Up to three controls were selected for each case. A total of 108 cases and 228 matched controls participated in the study. Influenza vaccine exposure was determined on the basis of medical chart reviews and telephone interviews for those vaccinated outside the HMO. Odds ratios were calculated using conditional logistic regression stratified by matching variables and adjusted for family history, race and ethnicity, place of birth, Scandinavian ancestry, smoking, and marital status.

With a case definition based on the presence in the medical record of a physician's diagnosis of optic neuritis, the odds ratio for optic neuritis following influenza vaccination was 1.2 (95% CI 0.6-2.3). The authors concluded that the results did not support the hypothesis that influenza vaccine causes the development of optic neuritis. They cited as strengths of the study that it was a large population-based study, that recall bias was minimized by inclusion of recently diagnosed cases and use of medical records, and that the results were consistent with different case definitions.

TABLE 5 Exposure to Influenza Vaccines and Multiple Sclerosis Relapse

Citation	Design	Population	Assessment of Vaccine Exposure
Myers et al. (1977)	Randomized controlled trial	Patients with active or inactive multiple sclerosis (MS). Age range of subjects = 26-64 years. Vaccinated: 23 Placebo: 23 Untreated controls: 22 Patients from two Los Angeles MS clinics and from private practice of UCLA neurologist	Randomization to receive either 1976 influenza vaccine (bivalent, whole virus) or placebo (vaccine diluent) Patients with active and inactive MS randomized separately. Patients and physicians blinded to vaccination status. Active MS defined as relapse within previous 3 months or progressive deterioration over past 6 months.

Outcomes	Results	Comment	Contribution to Causality Argument

MS relapse
 	
Patients were evaluated by a neurologist at 3 weeks and 3 months after injection.
	Frequency of relapse within 3 months following injection
	
	Vaccine group: 4
	  Myelopathy: 3
	  Mild relapse: 3
	  Moderate relapse: 1
	  Relapse Rate: 0.5 case/ patient/year
	
	Placebo group: 4
	  Myelopathy: 3
	  Moderate relapse: 2
	  Severe relapse: 1
	  Relapse Rate: 0.5 case/ patient/year
	
	Untreated group: 4
	  Myelopathy: 1
	  Mild relapse: 4
	  Relapse Rate: 0.7 case/ patient/year
		Based on the similar relapse rates among the groups, the authors concluded that vaccination against influenza is safe for patients with MS.	The study provides evidence of no association between exposure to the influenza vaccines and relapse of MS in adults.

continues

TABLE 5 Continued

Citation	Design	Population	Assessment of Vaccine Exposure
Bamford et al. (1978)	Cohort	127 MS clinic patients. Ages of subjects were not reported. Vaccinated: 65 Unvaccinated: 62 Arizona MS clinic	Vaccinated patients elected to receive bivalent influenza vaccine in November or December 1976.

Outcomes	Results	Comment	Contribution to Causality Argument
New or recurrent neurologic symptoms or increase in rate of deterioration observed during the month following vaccination. Vaccinated patients were asked about any allergic or toxic reactions to the vaccine.	*Frequency of outcomes:* Vaccinated group: Systemic toxic reactions: 2 Onset of neurologic symptoms: 1 Increased severity of preexisting dysfunction: 1 Episodes of deterioration: 0.031 per patient-month of exposure Unvaccinated group: New neurologic symptoms: 2 Increased disability: 2 Episodes of deterioration: 0.032 per patient-month of exposure	The authors noted that the occurrence of symptoms was similar to findings from other studies and concluded that the vaccine did not seem to adversely affect individuals already diagnosed with MS. Limitations include: No statistical tests were reported; the short time frame (four weeks) between vaccination and reporting of outcome; and patients self-selecting to receive the vaccine and self-reporting outcomes.	The study provides evidence of no association between exposure to influenza vaccines and relapse of MS; weaknesses in the study limit its contribution to the causality argument.

continues

TABLE 5 Continued

Citation	Design	Population	Assessment of Vaccine Exposure
Miller et al. (1997)	Random-ized con-trolled trial	104 patients with relapsing-remitting MS. Ages of subjects were not reported. Vaccinated: 49 Placebo: 54 Patients from 5 MS centers in Northeastern U.S.	Randomization to receive either 1993 vaccine or placebo. Each center had its own randomization process. Both investigators and subjects were blinded to vaccination status.
Mokhtarian et al. (1997)	Con-trolled trial	19 MS patients. Age range = 23-60 years. Vaccinated: 11 Placebo: 8 Vaccinated healthy controls: 9 New York	Vaccinated participants received either 1993 trivalent influenza vaccine prepared by a single manufacturer or placebo (vaccine diluent). No randomization procedures were reported. Basis for assignment to vaccine or placebo group unclear.

Outcomes	Results	Comment	Contribution to Causality Argument
MS exacerbations within 28 days or within 6 months after vaccination. Patients examined by a neurologist. MS exacerbation defined as increase of at least 0.5 on expanded disability status scale (EDSS), of at least one grade on scores of two or more of the Kurtzke functional system scores (FSS), or of two grades on one of the FSS. Changes persisted for more than 24 hours (or more than 48 hours after a fever).	*Exacerbations after 28 days:* Non-significant difference in exacerbations between vaccine group and placebo group. (Fisher's exact test) *Exacerbations after 6 months:* Non-significant difference in exacerbations between vaccine group and placebo group (chi-square analysis) Mean change in disability was not significant between two groups (t-test)	The authors concluded that influenza vaccinations did not appear to be associated with an increased risk of MS relapse.	The study provides evidence of no association between exposure to influenza vaccines and relapse of MS.
Exacerbation of MS. Neurologist examined participants before inoculation and after inoculation at 4 weeks, then followed for 6 months. Patients asked to report clinical exacerbations of MS.	*Frequency of Exacerbations:* Vaccine group, MS patients: 3 exacerbations at 19, 98, and 177 days after vaccination. Placebo group, MS patients: 2 exacerbations at 22 and 43 days after vaccination No significant difference in EDSS at the beginning and end of the study for either the influenza- or placebo-vaccinated groups.	Authors noted that late exacerbations in the influenza vaccinated MS patients may have been unrelated to vaccination. They concluded that the study provided no indication that influenza vaccine was associated with exacerbation of MS in patients with an EDSS of less than 6.5. Authors noted study limitations, including small sample size and lack of formal statistical analysis.	The study provides evidence of no association between exposure to influenza vaccines and relapse of MS in adults; weaknesses in the study limit its contribution to the causality argument.

continues

TABLE 5 Continued

Citation	Design	Population	Assessment of Vaccine Exposure
Confavreux et al. (2001)	Case-cross-over	643 subjects with MS (definite or probable) and at least one index relapse. Mean age = 37/39 years (+/- 10-11). *Cases:* Patients who experienced an index relapse between 1/93–12/97, with previous 12 months being relapse-free. *Controls:* Same patients during the first 8 months of the 12-month period before the index relapse. European Database for Multiple Sclerosis Network; France, Spain, Switzerland.	Vaccination history collected from study subjects by telephone interview and confirmed with written medical documentation. Vaccines received during study period included influenza, Hep A, HepB, tetanus, typhoid, yellow fever, typhoid-paratyphoid, tetanus-poliovirus, tetanus-diphtheria, or tetanus-poliovirus-diphtheria.

Outcomes	Results	Comment	Contribution to Causality Argument
Relapse between 1/93–12/97 in patients with diagnosed MS.

Neurologist categorized relapse as either definite, probable, or possible. Confirmed by neurologist through review of medical files. | *Relative Risk of relapse within 2 months after vaccination (95% CI):*

Influenza vaccine = 1.08 (0.37-3.10)

Any vaccine: 0.71 (0.40-1.26) | Authors noted that findings were inconclusive with regard to long-term risks. Study limitations included lower power for assessing risks associated with specific vaccines, exclusion of patients with frequent or minor relapses, and assumptions of constancy of vaccine exposure and equality of risk after each exposure. Study strengths included limited confounding by nature of study design, high response rates and validation of vaccine exposures, limited recall bias, and results unaffected by change in length of effect periods. The committee notes that the 1.08 RR may reflect not only the effect of the influenza vaccine on MS relapse, but also the adverse effect of acute illness. | The study suggests no association between exposure to influenza vaccines and MS relapse. |

continues

TABLE 5 Continued

Citation	Design	Population	Assessment of Vaccine Exposure
Sibley et al. (1976)	Uncontrolled observational	93 MS patients who received influenza vaccine, 1962-1975. Ages of subjects were not reported. MS Clinic at the University of Arizona Medical Center	Vaccination histories obtained from medical records. Patients received polyvalent influenza vaccine between 1962-1975.
De Keyser et al. (1998)	Uncontrolled observational study	233 MS patients Primary progressive MS: 53 Relapsing MS: 180 Mean age = 44 years Patients registered in the Groningen MS DataBank, Netherlands	Patients were asked if they received influenza vaccine in autumn 1996 (trivalent product for the 1996-1996 influenza season).

Outcomes	Results	Comment	Contribution to Causality Argument
Exacerbation of MS symptoms. Medical records were reviewed to obtain information on subsequent deterioration of MS symptoms following vaccination. Patients were also interviewed about reactions to vaccination (e.g., fever, allergic reactions, headaches) that suggested an attack of MS. Neurological symptoms occurring within one month after vaccination were considered vaccine-related.	*Percentage of reactions:* Vaccine-related: 19% Observed rate of relapse of 1 attack in 93 patient-months of observation was less than expected for the natural course of the disease (4.5 exacerbations per month).	No comparison control group. No formal statistical analyses conducted.	The study design limits the study's contribution to the causality argument.
Patients were asked form of MS (primary progressive or relapsing), severity of disability, duration of disease, and if they had experienced worsening or exacerbations of MS in the 6 weeks following influenza vaccination. Patients were also asked if they had experienced influenza illness.	*Number vaccinated:* Primary progressive group: 24 Relapsing MS patients: 70 Exacerbations: 4 (5%) experienced exacerbations in 6 weeks after vaccination (p<0.0001). *Number reporting illness:* Primary progressive group: 4 Relapsing MS patients: 36 Exacerbations: 12 (33%) experienced exacerbations after influenza illness.	No comparison control group. Patients reporting influenza illness may have had a disease other than influenza.	The study design limits its contribution to the causality argument.

continues

TABLE 5 Continued

Citation	Design	Population	Assessment of Vaccine Exposure
Salvetti et al. (1995; 1997)	Case series	6 MS patients Age range = 25-40 years	Received influenza vaccine.
VAERS	Case-series	Case reports submitted to VAERS between July 1990 and March 2003.	Receipt of influenza vaccine as reported to VAERS.

Outcomes	Results	Comment	Contribution to Causality Argument
Increase in clinical disease activity during the year following vaccination. Gd-MRI assessment 1 day before and 15 and 45 days after vaccination.	One patient experienced considerable worsening with a shift from relapsing-remitting to progressive MS during the post-vaccination year. Gd-MRI signs of disease activity at day 15 after vaccination.	Small number of cases studied. Patient with worsening condition experienced extremely active disease during previous year. Gd-MRI must be interpreted with caution.	The study design limits its contribution to the causality argument.
Multiple sclerosis; cases identified on the basis of inclusion of MS as an indexing term. Cases were excluded if they also included Guillain-Barré as an indexing term.	Number of MS reports 24	The analytical value of data from passive surveillance systems is limited by such problems as underreporting, lack of detail, inconsistent diagnostic criteria, and inadequate denominator data (Ellenberg and Chen, 1997; Singleton et al., 1999). Information did not indicate whether reports concerned onset of MS or relapses.	The nature of VAERS reports limits their contribution to the causality argument.

TABLE 6 Evidence Table: Exposure to Influenza Vaccines and Incident MS

Citation	Design	Population	Assessment of Vaccine Exposure
DeStefano et al. (2003)	Case-Control	332 cases 722 matched controls Subjects were divided into the following age groups (years): <18, 18-30, 31-40, >40 *Cases:* (1) Physician diagnosis of MS on medical records or (2) diagnosis by specialist or (3) meeting International Panel criteria for MS. *Controls:* Up to three per case, matched according to year of HMO enrollment, age, and sex. (Vaccine Safety Datalink, U.S.)	Receipt of influenza vaccine before index date. Influenza vaccine exposure was determined on the basis of medical chart reviews and telephone interviews for those vaccinated outside the HMO. *Cases:* 16.6% received influenza vaccination before the index date. *Controls:* 18.6% were vaccinated.
Kurland et al. (1984)	Uncontrolled Observational Study	U.S. Army personnel from 1975-1979 (765,000-779,000 active duty personnel) *Exposed* 85% received the swine influenza vaccine Cases occurring in 1976 compared to cases occurring in 1975-1979	Influenza vaccine given to all active duty military personnel in October. New recruits are administered the vaccine when they begin service.

Outcomes	Results	Comment	Contribution to Causality Argument
Physician diagnosis of MS in medical record. Potential cases found from screening outpatient and discharge data from three HMOs for 1995-1999. Of 556 cases confirmed by chart review, 332 had MS, were contacted, and participated in telephone interview.	*Adjusted OR (95% CI):* Medical diagnosis: 0.7 (0.5-1.1) International Panel criteria: 1.0 (0.6-1.4) *Adjusted OR (95%CI)* *using alternate case* *definitions and combining* *MS and optic neuritis (ON)* Specialist diagnosis: 0.9 (0.6-1.3) *Adjusted OR (95%CI) for* *timing of influenza* *vaccination and risk of* *demyelinating disease* *(MS and ON combined)* <1 yr before index date: 0.8 (0.5-1.4) 1-5 yrs: 1.1 (0.7-1.7) > 5 yrs: 0.6 (0.3-1.1)	Authors cite study's strengths as including study sample from large HMO population, minimizing recall bias by using recently diagnosed cases, using medical records to establish timing of MS onset and of vaccination, and consistent results using different case definitions. Limitations include reliance on information from subjects who were vaccinated outside HMO. Exclusion of self-reported date had little effect on results.	The study suggests no association between exposure to influenza vaccines and incident MS in adults.
New diagnosis of MS.	*Number of incident MS* *cases:* Average per calendar year: 6.55 1976, final quarter: 5 1977 first quarter: 6 7 quarters preceding 1976: 57 Final quarter of 1976 and next 6 quarters: 45	The authors interpret the data as indicating that the 1976 influenza vaccine did not affect the immediate or longer-term risk of developing MS among U.S. Army personnel.	The study design limits the study's contribution to the causality argument.

Other Information: Passive Surveillance Data, Case Reports

Information was presented to the committee that from January 1990 through March 2003, VAERS had received 26 reports of optic neuritis[8] following influenza vaccination (Haber, 2003). Case reports of optic neuritis and related conditions following influenza vaccination have also appeared in the published literature (Kawasaki et al., 1998; Ray and Dreizin, 1996; Sibley et al., 1976.

Causality Argument

With a single epidemiologic study available (DeStefano et al., 2003) (see Table 7), **the committee concludes that the evidence is inadequate to accept or reject a causal relationship between influenza vaccines and optic neuritis in adults.** VAERS data and case reports have limited value in assessments of causality. Because the available studies that examined optic neuritis did not specifically include children, the committee could not reach a conclusion on causality in the children's age group, but also could not clearly define the lower age limit for its conclusion in adults.

Other Demyelinating Neurological Conditions

Several case reports have been published mentioning the occurrence of other neurological disorders (e.g., acute disseminated encephalomyelitis, transverse myelitis) after influenza vaccination (Saito et al., 1980; Yahr and Lobo-Antunes, 1972; Bakshi and Mazziotta, 1996; Larner and Farmer, 2000). Other neurological conditions were reported from the surveillance system set-up during the 1976 National Influenza Immunization Program, but the data were not sufficient to assess causality (Retailliau et al., 1980). No other epidemiological studies were identified. Based on the nature of case reports and the paucity of epidemiological data, **the committee concludes that the evidence is inadequate to accept or reject a causal relationship between influenza vaccines and other demyelinating neurological disorders.**

Children and Influenza Vaccines

Influenza vaccine is generally administered to adults, and relatively few studies have reported data concerning any neurological complications observed in children. Currently, ACIP encourages influenza immunization for healthy children aged 6-23 months when feasible (CDC, 2003d). A recommendation for

---

[8]The outcome category "optic neuritis" was based on indexing terms (COSTART) found in the reports, not diagnostic or medical coding terms. Reports were counted as optic neuritis if they did not also mention GBS.

universal routine influenza immunization in that age group may be made in the near future (CDC, 2003d). Given concerns that demyelinating neurological disorders might follow receipt of influenza vaccines, the committee describes the relevant data in children, specifically focusing on the age group 6-23 months .

Both GBS and MS are rare in children, adding to the difficulty of studying any risk that might be associated with influenza vaccination. Schonberger and colleagues (1979), in their study of GBS and the swine influenza vaccine, reported two cases of GBS occurring in vaccinated children in the age group 0–17 years, compared with 120 cases occurring during the same period (October 1, 1976–January 31, 1977) in unvaccinated children. Looking only at cases of GBS that occurred within 6 weeks of vaccination, they calculated attack rates of 1.1 cases per million population per month for the vaccinated children and 0.46 for the unvaccinated children (RR = 2.4, 95% CI 0.4-16.2). However, because of the small number of cases and vaccinations in children, the authors noted that the risk estimates for children were less precise than those for adults.

In their data for Ohio, Marks and Halpin (1980) calculated a rate of 2.8 cases of GBS per million (1 case) for swine influenza vaccinees in the age group 0–24 years group compared with a rate of 2.4 per million (11 cases) for persons in that age group who had not been vaccinated (RR = 1.2, reported as not significant based on χ^2 test). It was not possible for the committee to determine which (if any) of the Ohio cases occurred in children.

Breman and Hayner (1984) examined the incidence of GBS in Michigan from July 1, 1976, through April 30, 1977. They found no cases of GBS among 99,263 children (ages 0–17 years) who received swine influenza vaccine in 1976. Among the 2.8 million children who were not vaccinated, 16 cases of GBS were found, an incidence rate of 0.13 per million person-weeks. By comparison, the incidence of GBS among unvaccinated adults was 0.36 per million person-weeks. Of the 16 children who had GBS, 13 had onset during the period January–April 1977, including 6 with a recent respiratory infection.

The committee also found a limited number of more recent reports (France, 2003; Neuzil et al., 2001; Gonzalez et al., 2000; Piedra et al., 1993) on studies of the safety of trivalent inactivated influenza vaccines in children. However, these studies provided no basis for assessing causal associations with the neurological conditions being considered in this report. Three studies (Neuzil et al., 2001; Gonzalez et al., 2000; Piedra et al., 1993) that examined the safety of influenza vaccines did not report any neurological reactions after receipt of influenza vaccines and did not report data specifically in the age group 6-23 months. Moreover, the small number of subjects in these studies limited their ability to detect diseases such as GBS and MS, which are rare in children. France (2003) reported to the committee on unpublished data from a VSD-based study. He and his colleagues have found no cases of MS or other demyelinating disorders in children after a review of medical records for specific ICD-9 diagnostic codes.

TABLE 7 Evidence Table: Exposure to Influenza Vaccines and Optic Neuritis

Citation	Design	Population	Assessment of Vaccine Exposure
DeStefano et al. (2003)	Case-Control	108 cases 228 matched controls Subjects were divided into the following age groups (years): <18, 18-30, 31-40, >40 *Cases:* Physician diagnosis of optic neuritis (ON) in medical records or diagnosis by specialist. *Controls:* Up to 3 per case, matched according to year of HMO enrollment, age, and sex. (Vaccine Safety Datalink, United States).	Receipt of influenza vaccine before index date. Influenza vaccine exposure was determined on the basis of medical chart reviews and telephone interviews for those vaccinated outside the HMO.
VAERS	Case-series	Case reports submitted to VAERS between July 1990 and March 2003.	Receipt of influenza vaccine as reported to VAERS

Outcomes	Results	Comment	Contribution to Causality Argument
Physician diagnosis of ON in medical record. Potential cases found by screening outpatient and discharge data from three HMOs for 1995–1999. Of 556 cases confirmed by chart review,108 had ON, were contacted, and participated in telephone interview.	*Adjusted OR (95%CI):* 1.2 (0.6–2.3)	Authors cite study's strengths as including study sample from large HMO population, minimized recall bias by using recently diagnosed cases, use of medical records to establish timing and onset of ON and of vaccination, and consistent results using different case definitions.	The study suggests no association between exposure to influenza vaccines and first episode of ON in adults.
Optic neuritis; cases identified on the basis of inclusion of optic neuritis as indexing term. Cases were excluded if they also included Guillain-Barré as an indexing term.	*Number of optic neuritis reports:* 26	The analytical value of data from passive surveillance systems is limited by such problems as underreporting, lack of detail, inconsistent diagnostic criteria, and inadequate denominator data (Ellenberg and Chen, 1997; Singleton et al., 1999).	The nature of VAERS reports limits their contribution to the causality argument.

The published reports concerning the 1976 swine influenza vaccine and GBS (Schonberger et al., 1979; Marks and Halpin, 1980; Breman and Hayner, 1984) and the reports on the safety of trivalent inactivated influenza vaccine in children (Neuzil et al., 2001; Gonzalez et al., 2000; Piedra et al., 1993) did not directly examine the relationship between influenza vaccines and demyelinating neurological disorders in children. These studies use a broad and varied definition of "children," and the small number of children in the studies limit the ability to detect rare neurological outcomes, such as GBS and MS. The committee reviewed one unpublished study that reported no cases of MS or other demyelinating disorders in children (France, 2003), but the unpublished nature of the study and the small number of cases limit its use in assessing causality. No published studies directly examined receipt of influenza vaccines and the occurrence of demyelinating neurological disorders in children. Thus, based on the lack of direct published evidence on influenza vaccines and demyelinating neurological disorders in children, especially those aged 6-23 months, **the committee concludes that there is no evidence bearing on a causal relationship between influenza vaccines and demyelinating neurological disorders in children aged 6-23 months.**

Biological Mechanisms

Although biological data do not provide an independent basis for evaluating causality, they can help validate epidemiologically based conclusions that are for or against causal associations. Such data can also guide further investigation when epidemiological evidence is inconclusive. In its assessment of the possibility of a relationship between influenza vaccines and neurological complications, the committee hypothesized two general ways vaccine could lead to neurological complications: immune-mediated processes and neurotoxic effects.

Before discussing these mechanisms, there is the issue of year-to-year variability in influenza vaccine and the role this could play in explaining variability in adverse effects (e.g. a causal association with the 1976 vaccine and no causal association with other influenza vaccines). The antigenic drifts that lead to the requirement for yearly influenza vaccination could influence the variability in adverse event profile. It is well known that other vaccine viruses show markedly different adverse effect profiles with only small differences between the viruses. For example, the Urabe strain mumps virus vaccine (never used in the United States) was causally associated with aseptic meningitis, but the Jeryl Lyn strain (used in the U.S. vaccine) is not (IOM, 1994a). The Sabin type 3 polio vaccine virus' neurovirulence changes dramatically with just a very few point mutations (Evans et al., 1985). The influenza A strains vary remarkably in their ability to grow in different species, different cell lines, and in eggs. Stimulation of interferon is very limited by some strains and quite prominent by others. Thus, it is not necessarily surprising that even closely related influenza viruses, including killed vaccine strains, could be associated with very different adverse effect profiles.

Immune-mediated Processes

There is considerable evidence that the demyelination in the PNS or CNS that occurs in diseases like GBS and MS is the result of inflammatory, immune-mediated processes (Noseworthy et al., 2000; Stuve and Zamvil, 1999; Waubant and Stuve, 2002). The concern addressed in this report is that, under certain circumstances, the initiation of the process that produces demyelination might be related to the activation of the immune system in response to influenza vaccination.

In trying to assess whether and how influenza vaccines might have such effects, the committee reviewed biological evidence, summarized below, regarding mechanisms by which immune responses to infection or vaccination might, in theory, play a role in triggering demyelination. The committee also reviewed evidence from animal models as to whether influenza vaccines might be expected to induce relevant immune-system responses. Because the influenza vaccine uses antigens that are produced by the influenza viruses, evidence regarding neurological complications following influenza infections was also considered relevant.

Theoretical Mechanisms for Infection-Induced Immune-Mediated Neurological Injury. Infection can induce immune-mediated tissue injury. In most cases, this injury is short-lived and resolves as the immune system eliminates active infection. The injury is a consequence of the immune response to the foreign invader, and when the invader is eliminated, the damaging immune process ceases. In some diseases, however, infection appears to induce an injurious immune response in the form of T and B cells that are directed, at least in part, against self-antigens. This autoimmune injury must be distinguished from immune-mediated injury that results from persistent but undetected infection. If the infectious agent was not detected, ongoing immune-mediated responses to that agent and the resulting injury of host tissues could be interpreted as auto-immunity, when in fact the immune response was directed against the foreign microbe and not against self.

The two major mechanisms proposed to account for the activation of self-reactive T and B cells and the induction of autoimmunity by infection are molecular mimicry and bystander activation (Albert and Inman, 1999; Bach and Chatenoud, 2001; Benoist and Mathis, 2001; Davidson and Diamond, 2001; Marrack et al., 2001; Regner and Lambert, 2001; Rose, 2001; Singh, 2000; Wucherpfennig, 2001; Zinkernagel, 2001). For a more extensive discussion of these mechanisms, see a previous report of this committee (IOM, 2002b).

Molecular mimicry is a mechanism by which an antigenic epitope from an infectious agent or other exogenous substance that is structurally similar to (mimics) an epitope of a self-molecule has the potential to trigger the activation of self-reactive, naïve T or B lymphocytes. Once activated, self-reactive T cells could expand in number and mature into effector (memory) T cells that have a lower threshold for activation by self-antigens. These cells would also gain the ability to migrate to specific tissues, produce additional mediators/cytokines, and mediate injury on contact with cross-reacting self-antigens. In addition, they would gain the potential to help B cells that are responding either to the same antigen as the T cells or to other self-antigens that are physically linked to it.

Bystander activation results when an infection creates environmental conditions that allow the activation of self-reactive T and B cells that are normally held in check. For example, tissue damage from an infection (or an inflammatory process) can lead to the liberation or exposure of host antigens in a context that allows for presentation to, activation of, and expansion of self-reactive lymphocytes.

Bystander activation does not require that antigens of the infectious agent be structurally similar to self-antigens. Instead, processes like the infection-induced death of host cells can result in the release of greater amounts of self-peptides or in the generation of novel self-peptides (i.e., novel or cryptic epitopes not normally found in the absence of the infection). At the same time, molecules derived from the infectious organism (and perhaps also from the necrotic host cells—e.g., heat-shock proteins) function as an adjuvant to help stimulate other components of the immune system to respond to the self-peptides.

Theoretical Mechanisms for Vaccine-Induced Immune-Mediated Neurological Complications. It is conceivable that vaccine antigens could mimic self (host), that stimulation from vaccines could trigger bystander activation just as an infectious organism does, and that either or both of these potentially damaging mechanisms could possibly lead to the development of central or peripheral demyelinating disease. There is no reason in theory why influenza virus antigens, or other substances in the vaccines (e.g., residual traces of constituents from the production process), could not function in this way. Thus, there is a theoretical basis for influenza vaccines to induce immune responses that could possibly lead to demyelination. As discussed in the subsequent section, however, the evidence in support of this theory is limited, and some is indirect.

Evidence from Animal Models for a Possible Role of Influenza Vaccines in Neurological Complications. The most studied animal model for GBS and its peripheral demyelination is experimental allergic neuritis (EAN), which has been best described in Lewis rats. EAN can be induced by active immunization with peripheral nerve myelin (as a homogenate of whole peripheral nerve tissue, peripheral myelin extracts, myelin proteins P2 and P0, or neuritogenic epitopes from P2) combined with complete Freund's adjuvant (Hahn, 1996; Vriesendorp, 1997). The Lewis rats develop progressive tail and limb paralysis about 10 days after immunization with myelin constituents, and histology demonstrates inflammation and demyelination of peripheral nerves.

In a 1983 report, Ziegler and colleagues described inducing an EAN-like disease in rabbits by injecting large doses of influenza vaccine combined with gangliosides (the major surface molecules in the PNS and CNS, expressed on myelinated neurons), cholesterol, and Freund's complete adjuvant. Indications of disease appeared at 21 to 56 days after inoculation. In addition to the PNS lesions characteristic of EAN, the spinal cords of some animals were affected. The EAN-like condition could be produced with vaccines containing swine influenza antigens and with vaccines with other influenza antigens. Regardless of the vaccine used, though, the inclusion of the gangliosides in the inoculation mixture was essential for induction of symptoms.

Another model of peripheral demyelination—experimental neuritis (EN)—also requires that a triggering agent, such as various viruses or antigens, be administered concomitantly with myelin tissue. In this model, the swine influenza vaccine was shown to trigger autoimmune responses and peripheral demyelination (Hjorth et al., 1984). The presence of the vaccine was important for the development of neuritis when low doses of nerve homogenate were injected. However, when high doses of nerve homogenate were used, the need for co-administration of swine influenza vaccine to elicit symptoms of disease was reduced.

For diseases that involve CNS demyelination, such as MS, the best-established animal model is experimental autoimmune encephalomyelitis (EAE)—a syndrome induced in susceptible strains of mice and rats. The inducing agent is usually immunization with myelin antigens or the transfer of T lymphocytes reactive against myelin proteins. Similarities between EAE models in animals and MS in humans include genetic susceptibility, greater female susceptibility, the clinical presentation, and the pathology. Studies of EAE offered no direct evidence concerning concerning influenza vaccine.

Other animal models for MS include demyelination induced by viral infections. Theiler's murine encephalomyelitis virus, for example, produces inflammatory demyelination of the spinal cord in mice. The effect appears to be mediated in part by T cells directed against viral antigens.

The similarities of EAN and EAE to the human demyelinating diseases GBS and MS, respectively, provide a strong indication that immunization with certain antigens can trigger autoimmune processes that produce demyelinating injuries. The committee found no evidence that exposure to influenza vaccines alone leads to EAN or EAE. But the studies of the EAN-like disease (Ziegler et al., 1983) and of EN (Hjorth et al., 1984) suggest that the vaccine acted as an adjuvant for immune responses to the accompanying neural tissue (similar to what might happen with bystander activation). It is uncertain, however, which components of the influenza vaccines—virus or virus subunits or contaminants from the manufacturing process (such as endotoxin)—contributed to the adjuvant effects. For a comparable mechanism to operate in the context of routine human use of influenza vaccine, some form of neural injury would have to be initiated by the immunization process (e.g., injuring a nerve while injecting the vaccine) to release neural antigens with which the vaccine would act as adjuvant.

The committee notes that no published follow-up studies could be found to confirm the 1983 report that influenza vaccines contributed to an EAN-like disease in rabbits or the 1984 report on the swine influenza vaccine in the EN model.

Evidence from Clinical Studies and *in vitro* Studies with Human Cells. There is inconclusive evidence that molecular mimicry between influenza vaccine glycoprotein antigens and PNS or CNS antigens plays a role in the pathogenesis of GBS, MS, or other neurological complications. As discussed above, immunization of rats with the myelin protein P2 or neuritogenic peptides derived from P2 can cause EAN, an experimental equivalent of GBS. Similarly, immunization of mice or rats with other myelin components can induce autoimmune demyelinating disease. This has caused some to ask whether influenza vaccines might contain myelin components or materials that mimicked myelin components.

An abstract published in 1981 but never followed by a peer-reviewed publication (Sheremata et al., 1981) suggested that influenza vaccines contained materials that cross-reacted with a polyclonal goat antiserum to bovine myelin P2 protein. However, the methods were not presented in the abstract, the specificity of the antiserum was not shown, and the actual data were not presented in a manner that could be independently reviewed. Brostoff and White (1982) tested nine lots of swine flu vaccine or combination swine flu and H3N2 influenza A vaccine from three manufacturers and were unable to detect P2 antigens by a sensitive radioimmunassay. Although the authors did not describe the relationship of the lots tested to the occurrence of GBS, the committee ascertained through CDC records that at least five of the nine lots tested were associated with GBS cases that occurred within 6 weeks of vaccination. Four of these lots were associated with between four and nine cases (Personal Communication, L. Schonberger, Centers for Disease Control and Prevention. September 4, 2003). However, the sensitivity of this assay for the detection of P2 proteins from species such as chicken, or proteins that might induce cross-reactive immunity in humans, is uncertain. Nonetheless, in the absence of any definitive reports on this issue, there is no evidence that influenza vaccines contain myelin components.

Shortly after it was found that T lymphocytes recognize short peptides bound to major histocompatibility molecules, which in humans are known as HLA molecules, several groups used computational methods to see if proteins in viruses, including influenza viruses, contained peptides that were homologous to peptides in myelin proteins. Similarities were found between peptides in proteins from multiple viruses, including influenza viruses, and myelin basic protein, or myelin P2 protein (Jahnke et al., 1985; Shaw et al, 1986; Weise and Carnegie, 1988). For a number of reasons, such reports do not provide evidence supporting the induction of autoimmunity to myelin through molecular mimicry.

First, these approaches only reveal hypothetical mimics. Even if the peptides were identical, which none of these were, amino acid identity is neither necessary nor sufficient to predict that they would induce cross-reactive autoimmunity to myelin in a physiological context. For example, the peptide might not be generated from the protein and presented on HLA molecules to T lymphocytes *in vivo*. Conversely and hypothetically, a peptide lacking sequence homology to a myelin protein could be generated and bind to HLA molecules in at-risk individuals in such a way that the HLA-peptide complex mimicked the structure of an HLA-myelin peptide complex. Thus, a peptide could lead to cross-reactive autoimmunity through molecular mimicry even though it had no sequence homology with peptides from myelin proteins.

Second, some of the homologies found were to the NS1 or NS2 proteins of influenza virus. NS1 and NS2 are non-structural proteins that accumulate in the nucleus of the infected cell but are not part of the mature influenza virus. Therefore any NS1 or NS2 produced during cultivation of vaccine-strain virus in chicken eggs should ordinarily be removed from the vaccine during purification. Whether NS1 or NS2 was actually present in influenza vaccine is unknown.

Finally, the committee was unable to identify published research further probing the implications and relevance for autoimmune demyelinating diseases of the sequence similarities between myelin and influenza proteins, including NS1 and NS2. Thus, there is no evidence supporting the notion of molecular mimicry between myelin proteins and components of influenza vaccines.

The use of embryonated chicken eggs in the production of virus for influenza vaccines raises the prospect of another possible source of antigens with structural similarities to PNS antigens. Chicken flocks are commonly infected asymptomatically with *Campylobacter jejuni*, with the bacterium spread in the fecal matter and sometimes found in eggs. Infection with *C. jejuni* is one of the most common precursors of GBS, and the surface antigens of GBS-associated *C. jejuni* strains have structural homology with human gangliosides. Specifically, sialic acid, a component of human gangliosides, is present on the outer core oligosaccharide (OS) portion of the lipopolysaccharide (LPS) of certain *C. jejuni* serotypes (Moran and Prendergast, 2001).

It is thought that the antiganglioside antibodies observed in some patients who develop GBS following *C. jejuni* infection may reflect molecular mimicry between peripheral nerve gangliosides and *C. jejuni* LPS. This hypothesis is supported by the finding that the most frequently isolated lipopolysaccharide/lipooligosaccharide of GBS-associated *C. jejuni* resemble GM1-and-GM2-structures (Moran et al., 2002). Anti-GM1 antibodies are the most frequently observed antibodies in GBS. In their review, Moran and colleagues (2002) also found that the molecular mimicry hypothesis was supported by serological studies, which demonstrated the binding of antiganglioside antibodies from GBS sera to surface epitopes of *C. jejuni* (GBS-associated serotypes).

Strong evidence supports molecular mimicry as a mechanism by which *C. jejuni* infection can lead to GBS. In the United States, nearly all GBS is of the demyelinating type, which is also true for GBS associated with *Campylobacter jejuni* and the GBS cases associated with "swine" flu vaccine (Personal Communication, A. Asbury, University of Pennsylvania, August 27, 2003). Although the use of eggs in the production of influenza vaccines appears to present the possibility that contamination with *C. jejuni* LPS/LOS could contribute to influenza vaccine-associated GBS, such contamination has not been demonstrated. However, influenza vaccines do contain endotoxin (lipopolysaccharides) in varying amounts (Geier et al., 2003; Hamada et al., 1989), which could contribute to bystander activation of the immune response, as described in the previous section. The microbes from which the lipopolysaccharides found in influenza vaccines are derived are unknown, so the possibility of *C.jejuni* LPS contamination of influenza vaccines cannot be excluded at the present time.

Effects of Influenza Virus Infection in Humans. When an infectious agent has been associated with a particular adverse health outcome, the possibility exists that a vaccine against that agent could have a similar effect. The primary manifestation of influenza infection is respiratory, but other symptoms may occur, such as myositis, rhabdomyolysis, and myoglobinuria.

Central or peripheral neurological manifestations are not generally a feature of influenza infection but are observed. Influenza-associated encephalitis/encephalopathy has been reported in certain populations—in particular, Japanese children—although a causal relationship has not been proven (Morishima et al., 2002; Sugaya, 2002). These cases primarily follow influenza A infection and are associated with unusually high morbidity and mortality rates. Encephalitis also occurs in association with influenza B infections, but much less frequently than with influenza A infections (Hochberg et al., 1975). Occurrence is also primarily in children (Newland et al., 2003). Rarely, acute encephalopathy occurs at the peak of influenza illness and may be fatal.

People with MS and their treating physicians have often worried that viruses, such as the influenza virus, may increase the risk of MS relapse. It is not prominent in the discussions of viral triggers for the onset of MS, however. In terms of the implications for risks that might be associated with influenza vaccines, one study has shown that the risk of relapse is substantially greater following influenza-like illness[9] than after influenza vaccination (De Keyser et al., 1998).

Studies of infections preceding GBS have found that influenza A and influenza B infection each preceded GBS in 1 percent of cases in the population studied, but not more frequently than in controls (Jacobs et al., 1998).

Known Effects of Other Vaccines. The evidence for causal associations between other vaccines and demyelinating diseases of either the CNS or PNS is mixed. A previous IOM committee found that the evidence favors acceptance of a causal relationship between tetanus-toxoid-containing vaccines and brachial neuritis, a peripheral nerve disorder possibly linked to immune-mediated reactions (IOM, 1994a). In addition, that same IOM committee concluded that the oral polio vaccine was associated with GBS (IOM, 1994a), but data (Kinnunen et al.,

---

[9]The authors noted that the self-reported influenza-like illness may have included some other etiologies other than influenza virus.

1998; Rantala et al., 1994) published after that report was issued suggested to some that the association was not causal (Sutter et al., 1999). Acute disseminated encephalomyelitis (ADEM), a demyelinating disease of the CNS, has been reported after vaccination with the Semple rabies vaccine (used outside the United States) and measles-containing vaccines (Stuve and Zamvil, 1999).

Conclusions Regarding Neurological Complications Resulting from Immune-Mediated Processes. In summary, there is a theoretical basis for mechanisms involving immune-mediated processes by which a vaccine could cause neurological complications, including a peripheral demyelinating disease like GBS or a central demyelinating disease like MS. There is no reason, in theory, why influenza vaccines could not operate in this way.

The following biological evidence relates to the theory that influenza vaccines could be associated with neurological complications:

• **Bystander activation.** Animal models (Hjorth et al., 1984; Ziegler et al., 1983) show that under contrived experimental conditions inoculation with influenza vaccines in combination with myelin antigens (as tissue or gangliosides) leads to demyelinating diseases similar in many respects to GBS. Animal models of MS-like CNS demyelination also exist but have not been linked to influenza viruses or vaccines. In models of peripheral demyelination (EAN-like disease and EN), influenza vaccines had adjuvant properties in the presence of neural antigens. For this model to operate during routine human use of influenza vaccine, neural injury would have to be initiated during the immunization process to release neural antigens with which the vaccine would act as adjuvant, or influenza vaccines would have to contain myelin (which has not been shown) or other components that mimic myelin.

• **Molecular mimicry.** Evidence related to molecular mimicry is mixed.

1. No direct evidence shows that influenza antigens or other vaccine components act as molecular mimics of self antigens in the nervous system. Although two older studies demonstrated similarities in amino acid sequences between the myelin protein P2 and the influenza A virus protein NS2, there is no evidence that this sequence similarity leads to structural similarity or that NS2 can elicit host autoantibodies. In addition, NS2 is not likely to be found in influenza vaccines.

2. A strong set of data indicate that *C. jejuni* antigens can trigger GBS through molecular mimicry. Influenza vaccines are made using viruses cultivated in eggs, and eggs can be contaminated with *C. jejuni*. Although the production of the 1976 swine influenza vaccine by four different manufacturers with four different proprietary seed viruses and different egg sources makes widespread *C. jejuni* contamination seem highly unlikely, the available evidence cannot exclude the possibility that *C. jejuni* antigens were present in the vaccines from all four manufacturers.

Additional but indirect evidence is provided by the causal relationship that has been found between brachial neuritis and vaccines other than those against influenza. Relationships between other vaccines and the neurological disorders of GBS and ADEM may also be causal, but evidence is not conclusive.

The committee concludes that there is weak evidence for biological mechanisms related to immune-mediated processes, including molecular mimicry and bystander activation, by which receipt of any influenza vaccine could possibly influence an individual's risk of developing the neurological complications of GBS, MS, or other demyelinating conditions such as optic neuritis.

Neurotoxic Effects

Neurotoxin

The FDA requires pre-release testing of samples of each lot of every vaccine used in the United States to ensure that the vaccine meets specifications for potency and purity. In theory, however, some component of influenza vaccines used in 1976 or certain other years might have had a direct neurotoxic effect that resulted in GBS in some recipients.

The essential component of influenza vaccines is the viral antigens, which are presented in the form of either whole inactivated virus particles (in older forms of the vaccine) or viral subunits. Influenza viruses themselves are not known to be toxic or to produce toxins, making it unlikely that the viral antigens in the vaccines would be toxic.

Questions have been raised, however, about the possibility that the thimerosal in certain vaccines recommended for children might have neurotoxic effects (see IOM, 2001b). Thimerosal is present as a preservative in multiple-dose vials of influenza vaccines. Single-dose vials that do not require a preservative may contain trace amounts of thimerosal remaining from the production process.

Thimerosal contains approximately 50 percent mercury by weight. At high doses, mercury and mercuric compounds—including thimerosal and its metabolite ethylmercury—are well-established neurotoxicants (ATSDR, 1999; EPA, 1997; NRC, 2000). Demyelinating disorders are not known to be caused by even high-dose mercury exposure.

Another possibility is that, in theory, influenza vaccines that have been epidemiologically associated with an increased risk of GBS—e.g., those produced in 1976—might have contained an unidentified contaminant with neurotoxic properties. The vaccines administered that year came from four different manufacturers and included whole- and split-virus products and monovalent and bivalent formulations. As discussed above, studies found no statistically significant difference among manufacturers or vaccine formulations in the increased risk for GBS.

In the absence of experimental or human evidence regarding the direct

neurotoxic effect of influenza vaccines, the committee concludes that this mechanism is only theoretical.

SIGNIFICANCE ASSESSMENT

Previous IOM vaccine safety studies focused on conclusions from causality assessments and recommendations for future research. The Immunization Safety Review Committee has been asked to also consider the public health response to the immunization safety concerns that it examines. In doing so, the committee examines the significance of the hypothesized associations between vaccines and adverse events in a broader social context—the context in which policy decisions must be made.

In the present case, the committee considered the significance of the concern that influenza vaccines might increase the risk of developing neurological complications such as GBS or MS. The scientific assessment provided support for a link between GBS and the 1976 influenza vaccines, but the evidence for other outcomes or for vaccines for other years was inadequate to support a conclusion or favored no association. No evidence was found between influenza vaccines and demyelinating neurological disorders in children. Vaccination plays a key role in efforts to reduce the annual impact of influenza infections, making it important that any vaccine-related risks be identified and evaluated. Reviewed here is the burden of illness (e.g., the severity, prognosis, and financial costs) associated with GBS, as well as that associated with influenza infections. Concerns about future influenza pandemics are also discussed. New types of influenza vaccines, expected to be available soon, and the risk-benefit communication of influenza immunization are described.

Disease Burden Associated with Guillain-Barré Syndrome

As described above, GBS is an acute, immune-mediated paralytic disorder of the PNS. It is characterized by rapidly progressive, ascending, and symmetric weakness, with loss of deep tendon reflexes, possible tingling in the feet and hands, and muscle aches (myalgia). Facial, oculomotor, oropharyngeal, and respiratory muscles may also be involved. Four different forms of the disease are recognized, distinguished in part by varying involvement of the motor and sensory nerve fibers (Asbury, 2000).

The severity of clinical defects typically peaks within the first 2 weeks after onset, but some deficits may continue to progress for 3 to 4 weeks. In the most serious cases, estimated at 20 percent of the total (Buzby et al., 1997), patients may require respiratory support. There is no known cure for GBS, but recovery can sometimes be aided by treatment, early in the course of the disease, with plasmapheresis or intravenous immunoglobulin. Most patients improve and return to normal functioning within 6 to 9 months, but some experience relapses or a prolonged disease course with residual neurological deficits, and death may occur. Because of its sudden and unexpected onset, GBS can be a devastating disorder (NINDS, 2001). Moreover, as noted above, recovery is not always timely. GBS patients not only face physical difficulties but emotional problems as well. It is often extremely challenging for patients to adjust to sudden paralysis and dependence on others for help with routine activities, and psychological counseling is often needed to help them adapt.

The incidence of GBS is usually estimated at 1 to 2 cases per 100,000 population per year (Hughes and Rees, 1997). This rate implies roughly 3,000 to 6,000 new cases a year in the United States, based on the current population of over 280 million. The causes of GBS are not fully understood, but a widely recognized risk factor, accounting for 20 to 40 percent of cases, is a prior infection with the foodborne pathogen *C. jejuni* (Buzby et al., 1997). In 1976, the incidence of GBS within 6 weeks influenza vaccination that was considered attributable to vaccination was estimated at 0.488 to 0.567 case per 100,000 vaccinations (Langmuir et al., 1984). For the 1992–1993 and 1993–1994 influenza seasons, an analysis suggested that vaccination may have been responsible for 0.11 case of GBS per 100,000 vaccinations (Lasky et al., 1998).

People of all ages can develop GBS, although incidence appears to be higher among adults than among children. From 2 to 5 percent of cases are fatal, with most deaths occurring among patients who require mechanical ventilation (Buzby et al., 1997; Sunderrajan and Davenport, 1985). The average cost of medical care and lost productivity for GBS has been estimated at $470,000 (1995 dollars) per case (Buzby et al., 1997).

Influenza Infections and Vaccination

Disease Burden

Influenza is a highly infectious viral illness that peaks in autumn and winter months in the United States. Frequent changes in the antigenic characteristics of the influenza viruses in circulation mean that many people in the population are susceptible to infection each year. Up to 20 percent of the population may be infected in a single year (Palese and Garcia-Sastre, 2002). Infection rates frequently exceed epidemic thresholds and occasionally reach pandemic levels.

The risk of serious illness and complications is greatest among very young children, persons aged 65 years or older, and individuals with underlying medical conditions. In the United States during the 1990s, an average of 36,000 influenza-associated deaths occurred each year (13.8 deaths per 100,000) (Thompson et al., 2003; CDC, 2003c), putting it among the leading causes of death. About 90 percent of these deaths were among persons aged 65 years or older. In nursing homes, 60 percent attack rates and 30 percent fatality rates have been recorded

(CDC, 2002a). Hospitalizations are necessary, however, across a broad age range. In children 4 years and younger, hospitalization rates ranged from about 100 per 100,000 in children without high risk medical conditions to approximately 500 per 100,000 in those who are at high risk. Children one year or younger had hospitalization rates similar to adults 65 years or over (CDC, 2003d). Data for the period 1969–1970 through 1994–1995 indicate that influenza epidemics were responsible for an average of 114,000 excess hospitalizations each year (excess of 49 pneumonia and influenza related hospitalizations per 100,000), with more than 57 percent occurring among persons younger than age 65 (CDC, 2003d).

Vaccination is the primary method for controlling influenza, but antiviral agents also have a role, primarily in treatment. Two related drugs, amantadine and rimantadine, can be used to prevent or treat infections by influenza A viruses but not influenza B viruses (Kilbourne and Arden, 1999). They act by interfering with the replication of the virus. Two newer antiviral products, zanamivir and oseltamivir, are effective against influenza A and B viruses in that they act as neuraminidase inhibitors. Some potentially serious side effects are associated with the amantadine drugs,[10] and drug-resistant organisms emerge rapidly, so use is generally reserved for controlling small outbreaks, such as in nursing homes, where many people could develop influenza illness and complications. Less is known about the safety and efficacy of the neuraminidase inhibitors (Hilleman, 2002).

The economic costs of influenza—for medical care and lost productivity— are substantial. CDC (2002a) reports that the total cost of a severe epidemic has been estimated to be $12 billion.

Influenza Vaccination

Vaccination is the most effective means of reducing the annual impact of influenza infections (CDC, 2002c). As previously described, the vaccine is updated each year to incorporate viral strains that closely match those in circulation. In the United States, inactivated influenza virus vaccines, using disrupted or split-virus formulations, are currently used (CDC, 2002a). Split-virus vaccines are associated with fewer local and systemic reactions,[11] especially in children, than

---

[10]The most frequent (5-10%) adverse reactions to amantadine are nausea, dizziness and insomnia. Less often, (1-5%) depression, anxiety and irritability, ataxia and other reactions can occur. Infrequently (0.1-1%), adverse events such as congestive heart failure, urinary retentions, dyspnea, optic nerve palsy and others occur. Rarely (< 0.1%), patients may have instances of convulsions, leucopenia, neutropenia, oculogyric episodes, and other adverse reactions (PDR, 2003).

[11]For example, some local adverse reactions include soreness, edema, tenderness, erythema, and inflammation at the vaccination site. Systemic reactions from the vaccine include fever, malaise, myalgia, arthralgia, chills, dizziness, headache, pruritus, rash, nausea, vomiting and diarrhea. Most of these systemic reactions occur in individuals who have had no exposure to the influenza virus antigens in the vaccine (PDR, 2003).

the previously produced whole-cell vaccines (Kilbourne and Arden, 1999). A live attenuated intranasal influenza vaccine was approved by the FDA in June 2003 for use in the United States in healthy individuals aged 5-49 years (DHHS, 2003). If the viral strains used to produce the vaccine are closely matched to the viral strains circulating during the influenza season, vaccination may prevent illness (although not necessarily infection) in 70 to 90 percent of healthy children as young as 6 months of age and healthy adults under age 65. (CDC, 2002b). Vaccination is only 30 to 40 percent effective in preventing illness in older and more frail individuals, but it is 50 to 60 percent effective in preventing hospitalization and 80 percent effective in preventing deaths (CDC, 2002a). CDC (2002b) notes conflicting evidence as to whether vaccination helps reduce the incidence of acute otitis media among young children. Cost-effectiveness studies show that vaccination reduces both the cost of medical care and the productivity losses associated with illness among the working-age population (Bridges et al., 2000; CDC, 2003d; Nichol, 2001).

Influenza vaccine must be given every year and is recommended for large segments of the population, making it the one of the most widely used vaccines in the United States. Nevertheless, despite evidence of the effectiveness of influenza vaccine, vaccination coverage levels are lower than what public health officials seek (CDC, 2003d). Estimates of vaccination coverage for 2001 were 67 percent for adults aged 65 years or older and 35 percent for adults aged 50–64 years. Estimates from 2000 showed that vaccination coverage was 29 percent among adults aged 18–64 years who had high-risk health conditions. Coverage among children for whom influenza vaccination is recommended are said to be low, but systematic data are not readily available.

Influenza vaccine is most effective when it is administered no more than 2 to 4 months before exposure to the virus (CDC, 2002a). In the United States, vaccination programs generally begin in October. In 2000 and 2001, manufacturers' production problems delayed the delivery of the vaccine (CDC, 2003d). Those problems were resolved for 2002, and CDC (2003d) reported that 95 million doses of vaccine were produced, of which 83 million were distributed (although not necessarily used). For 2003, the number of manufacturers supplying vaccine for the United States will decline from three to two.

Concerns about Pandemic Influenza

In addition to influenza's substantial toll every year, there is special concern about the impact of sporadic influenza pandemics—defined as disease epidemics that occur worldwide. Influenza pandemics are thought to arise because of a sudden shift in the influenza A subtype in circulation to one against which large segments of the population lack any immunity (e.g., from H1N1 to H2N2). With the last serious pandemic having occurred in 1968, influenza virologists agree that a new pandemic is overdue and imminent, but they are concerned that the global community is inadequately prepared (IOM, 2003; Webster, 1997; Webster, 2003). The 1918–1919 influenza pandemic had a profound impact. At least 20 million people died worldwide and probably 10 times more were affected (Webster, 1999). In the United States, this pandemic is believed to have taken the lives of at least 500,000 people and lowered the overall average life expectancy by almost 10 years (Palese and Garcia-Sastre, 2002). Less devastating pandemics occurred in 1957–1958 and 1968–1969 (see Table 8).

Future pandemics could arise from influenza viruses with novel surface antigens introduced into humans from animals. The 1957 and 1968 pandemic influenza strains were derived from reassortments of avian and human viral strains. The reassortment probably occurred in an intermediate host species, but that host is not known (Steinhauer and Skehel, 2002). Direct transmission from birds to humans is rare. Generally the directly transmitted viruses have low virulence except in a small subset of individuals, and transmissibility from person to person is limited (Hilleman, 2002). Direct transmission was suspected, however, when avian H9N2 infected two children in Hong Kong in 1999 (Lin et al., 2000).

New Vaccine Approaches

Since influenza vaccine was first introduced, the United States has relied on vaccine products based on inactivated influenza virus. In other countries, including Russia, vaccines that incorporate live attenuated influenza virus have been used for many years (Wareing and Tannock, 2001).

TABLE 8 Major Twentieth Century Influenza A Pandemics

Year	Virus Subtype	Deaths	Characteristics
1918–1919	A H1N1	United States: >500,000 Worldwide: 20–50 million	Majority of individuals affected were young, healthy adults
1957–1958	A H2N2	United States: ≈70,000	First identified in China in late February 1957; reached US by June 1957
1968–1969	A H3N2	United States: ≈34,000	First detected in Hong Kong in early 1968; reached US later that year. H3N2 virus still circulates today.

SOURCE: Table adapted from information provided on CDC website. (CDC, 2003c).

The FDA recently approved a live attenuated intranasal influenza vaccine for use in the United States. The vaccine uses a cold-adapted influenza virus master strain into which the HA and NA genes of the current, circulating strains are incorporated. The vaccine is delivered intranasally and proliferates in the upper airways, where it stimulates mucosal antibodies and T-cell responses. The use of a cold adapted master strain means that replication of the live virus in the vaccine is restricted to the upper respiratory tract of humans because the vaccine-strain virus is unable to reproduce in the higher-temperature environment of the lower respiratory tract. Cold adaptation was achieved by propagation of the wild-type virus in chicken kidney cells at progressively lower temperatures to identify stable mutants that could grow at 25°C (Maassab and Bryant, 1999).

A primary concern about a live-virus influenza vaccine is the possibility that the vaccine-strain viruses could undergo genetic reassortment with nonhuman (e.g., avian or swine) strains and give rise to new, virulent strains to which the population would be susceptible (Beyer et al., 2002; Pfleiderer et al., 2001). This theoretical concern has not been borne out in clinical studies, and similar vaccines given to tens of millions of children in Russia have not produced any clinical evidence of live attenuated vaccines reverting to virulence (Belshe et al., 2002; Cha et al., 2000).

Research related to killed-virus vaccines is also continuing. For example, efforts are being made to develop techniques to grow influenza virus in mammalian cell culture instead of eggs (Halperin et al., 2002). Other studies are looking at the influenza virus's M2 protein as a possible vaccine antigen that could eliminate the need to formulate a new vaccine each year to respond to the antigenic drift or shift in the circulating viruses. M2 is highly conserved antigenically, and antibodies to M2 have been shown to be protective in mice (Neirynck et al., 1999). There is also interest in developing a DNA vaccine, and studies immunizing mice with recombinant plasmids bearing coding sequences for selected HA, NP, or M proteins have been promising (Fu et al., 1999; Okuda et al., 2001).

Another approach to influenza vaccination involves using *Escherichia coli* heat-labile toxin as an adjuvant, complexed with lecithin vesicles, to improve the immunogenicity of the inactivated trivalent vaccine (Palese and Garcia-Sastre, 2002). These "virosomal" vaccine preparations are given intranasally.[12]

---

[12]One virosomal influenza vaccine licensed for use in Switzerland in 2000 was withdrawn a year later because of unresolved concerns about an association between the vaccine and Bell's palsy (temporary facial paralysis) (Berna Biotech, 2002). The committee did not examine this vaccine because it was not used in the United States, it is no longer available in Switzerland, and no published study is available.

Influenza Immunization Risk-Benefit Communication

Factors that affect people's understanding of health risks and the options to reduce those risks include, for example, personal attributes (e.g., age, gender, ethnicity, etc.), beliefs about the disease and potential control options, attitudes about the source(s) of those controls, the risk and benefits attributed to the controls, and the trade-offs among the controls. In addition, heuristics, as well as societal and decision contexts, matter in vaccine decision making (e.g., Leask and Chapman, 1998; Bostrom, 1997). Although the impacts of these factors on vaccine decisions are not well understood and may vary somewhat by type of vaccine, it is clear that no one factor acts alone. Both individual and contextual factors are important to the individual's final decision about whether to get vaccinated or not. It is well known, however, that people often lack knowledge about disease processes and the safety and effectiveness of vaccines, and usually do not know what critical information they are lacking. Individuals may also underestimate the risk of the disease and overestimate risks of the vaccine and their own abilities to avoid getting the disease (e.g., Bostrom, 1997; Fischhoff et al, 2000).

In developing a risk communication strategy for a specific health decision, it is important then to know what key pieces are missing from people's cognitive frameworks about the decision and related issues, what they need to know to complete and/or correct their understandings, and what factors and contexts strengthen their abilities to make effective and personally meaningful decisions. As noted by Bostrom (1997), there are several health behavior models and theories that can be applied to vaccination issues. To date there has not been a comprehensive effort to organize current knowledge and evaluate these models and theories using the results for various populations. Knowledge of the key factors that predict and/or influence influenza vaccination decisions remains constrained, thereby limiting the basis on which sound risk communication strategies can be designed. A more comprehensive and cohesive understanding is needed to identify what elements are crucial to people's decision processes, how they relate those and tangential elements, what they include and/or relate incorrectly in their decision processes, and what elements they emphasize or de-emphasize inappropriately. Risk communication efforts will remain less than ideal as long as they are not based on a full, fundamental picture of what people believe they know, what they see as valid and rational control options, what they believe the consequences of those options are, why they view vaccine issues as they do, and how they assess the trade-offs between the options.

Influenza vaccination rates typically fall short of national goals, particularly among susceptible subpopulations such as the elderly and disadvantaged. Several studies have been conducted recently to develop insights into the barriers and incentives that may affect immunization rates (CDC, 1999; CDC, 2003b; Zimmerman et al., 2003b). Societal contexts, influences of the mass media, and cognitive and motivational biases have been investigated.

People who were more likely to receive the influenza vaccine were found in these studies to be more likely to believe that:

- Getting vaccinated is a wise decision, a good habit.
- The recommendations of their doctors, relatives, or friends are important.
- The vaccine is effective in preventing influenza.
- Medicare will cover the costs.
- Avoiding getting influenza is important.
- They are at risk for getting the disease.
- Unvaccinated people will contract influenza.

People who did not get vaccinated had beliefs that differed from those who became vaccinated. Some of the key beliefs among non-vaccinees were:

- They are not at risk for influenza.
- The vaccine is not for them; it is for old, weak, or sick people.
- The vaccine causes influenza.
- The vaccine causes side effects.
- They had bad reactions to influenza vaccinations in the past.
- They do not need to be vaccinated.
- The vaccine will not prevent influenza.

Potential vaccine recipients have been found to have incomplete or incorrect knowledge about:

- The nature of influenza as a disease process (e.g., some believe it is part of spectrum of diseases that begins with the common cold and ends with pneumonia),
- the severity of the complications that may arise from influenza,
- the degree to which individual actions (e.g., hand washing, taking vitamins, etc.) can reduce the risk of getting the disease,
- the unique role of the vaccine as a preventive measure, and
- the health impacts and side effects related to the influenza vaccine.

In several studies, the most important source of vaccination information has been found to be health care providers, but physicians do not always recommend that their elderly patients receive the influenza vaccine, either in conjunction with or without the pneumococcal vaccine (CDC, 1999; CDC, 2003b; Zimmerman et al., 2003a,b).

Zimmerman and colleagues (2003a) studied the beliefs and attitudes of the same elderly people in vaccine supply-rich and supply-limited periods. They found shifts in the participants' attitudes and contexts. For example, during the vaccine shortage period the participants reported more doubts and concerns about the vaccine (including safety, efficacy, and side effects issues); declines in physicians' and friends' recommendations to get vaccinated; less concern about unvaccinated people getting ill; and fewer concerns that other family members would contract influenza if one person got it. These changes may have led potential vaccinees to further underestimate the risk of getting influenza and thus their need for vaccination.

CDC (2003b) also examined physicians' views about the influenza and pneumococcal vaccines. The participating physicians saw these vaccinations as an important patient service, demonstrated that they were knowledgeable about the vaccines, and said they wanted more involvement of their office managers in promoting the vaccinations. However, the physicians had little knowledge of the costs of the vaccinations and believed that people who were in the habit of visiting a doctor were more likely to be vaccinated.

These recent studies show that modifications to current influenza risk communication programs would be beneficial. People need more appropriate contexts; information that is relevant to their cultural, societal, and personal circumstances; and materials in a language they can understand. An effective communication strategy must not only simplify and summarize key information, but also ensure that the needs of a variety of at-risk populations are met. Frequently, this must be done through carefully tailored methods and messages for each group.

Conclusions

Influenza vaccine is an essential tool for reducing the substantial burden of morbidity and mortality associated with influenza infections each year. Not only is the yearly disease toll high, but the prospect of an influenza pandemic is a serious concern to many. Because the vaccine is used so widely, and may be recommended for regular administration to young children, the possibility of vaccine-related adverse events must be given serious consideration. But although it is important to fully understand any risk for GBS or other neurological complication that might be associated with influenza vaccination, it is also important that this be appropriately weighed against the sizable burden of illness associated with influenza infections.

In its scientific assessment, the committee found support for a causal association between the vaccine used in 1976 and GBS. But it found no support for an association with relapses of MS, and inconclusive evidence regarding influenza vaccines used in other years and other neurological conditions. The committee found no evidence bearing on a causal relationship between influenza vaccines and demyelinating neurological disorders in children aged 6-23 months. GBS is a serious condition, but it is rare and the additional risk related to vaccination in 1976 translated into fewer than 6 cases per million vaccinee (Langmuir et al., 1984). By contrast, influenza contributes to an annual average of 13.8 deaths per

100,000 (36,000 deaths, majority are 65 years of age or older) and to an annual excess of 49 pneumonia and influenza related hospitalizations per 100,000 (114,000 hospitalizations) (Thompson et al., 2003; Simonsen et al., 2000).

RECOMMENDATIONS FOR PUBLIC HEALTH RESPONSE

The committee's charge includes making recommendations regarding a broad range of actions, including potential policy reviews, research needs, and changes in communication to the public and to health care providers about issues of vaccine safety.

Policy Review

Despite evidence favoring a causal association between GBS and the influenza vaccines used in 1976, the committee sees no evidence regarding more recent influenza vaccines that would warrant a review of current influenza immunization policies. Vaccination against influenza remains an essential component of efforts to reduce the substantial morbidity and mortality associated with influenza infections.

The committee does not recommend a policy review of the recommendations for influenza vaccination by any of the national or federal vaccine advisory bodies on the basis of concerns about neurological complications. Current and future immunization policies should continue to reflect the benefits of influenza vaccination.

Research

The evidence reviewed by the committee does not support a causal association between influenza vaccines and MS relapses and is inconclusive on some other outcomes, but it does support an association between GBS and the influenza vaccines used in 1976 (i.e., whole- and split-virus products formulated as monovalent or bivalent vaccines). Although the 1976 vaccines are no longer in use, experience with them should not be ignored because the mechanism by which they contributed to GBS remains unclear. With a vaccine as widely used as influenza vaccine, the committee considers it important to pursue research and research-related activities aimed at ensuring that any risk of GBS or other neurological complications is minimized.

Surveillance and Epidemiologic Studies

Influenza vaccine is not only widely used but is recommended for even wider use than is routinely achieved. In addition, there are expectations that recommended use will be extended to include all children aged 6–23 months.

Even though use of the vaccine generally appears to pose minimal risk of adverse neurological events, the strong association between the 1976 vaccine and GBS points to the need for appropriate vigilance through adequate surveillance systems and for better tools to support studies of rare adverse events.

Currently, ACIP recommends annual influenza vaccination for any person aged 6 months or older who is at increased risk for complications from influenza (CDC, 2003d). The 2002 ACIP recommendations note that "because young, otherwise healthy children are at increased risk for influenza-related hospitalizations, influenza vaccination of healthy children aged 6–23 months is encouraged when feasible" (CDC, 2003d). But the ACIP, the American Academy of Pediatrics, and the American Academy of Family Physicians recognize that a full recommendation for annual vaccinations of all children aged 6–23 months cannot be made until certain issues are addressed (CDC, 2003d). Important among these is educating parents and providers regarding the impact of influenza infections in children and the risks and benefits of vaccination. Routine vaccination of children, some of whom may require two doses of vaccine within a season, will require the development of strategic plans to ensure efficient delivery of services within a limited time each year. Issues regarding vaccination costs and reimbursement policies must also be addressed. A recommendation for annual vaccinations of all children aged 6–23 months could be made in the near future (CDC, 2003d). In preparation for this change in influenza immunization practices, **the committee recommends increased surveillance of adverse events associated with influenza vaccination of children, with particular attentiveness to detecting and assessing potential neurological complications. Enhanced surveillance should be in place before an ACIP recommendation is implemented for universal annual influenza vaccination of young children.**

Better methods are needed to identify and assess risks for rare outcomes such as the neurological complications considered in this report. The scale of the 1976 vaccination program—almost 45 million people vaccinated within 2.5 months— helped make detection of the link with GBS feasible. CDC's Vaccine Safety Datalink program offers a valuable means of assembling systematic population-based data on vaccination and medical histories. Nevertheless, it may not cover a large enough population to successfully investigate concerns about some rare adverse events. Moreover, in the context of influenza vaccines, which are still given primarily to adults, the committee learned at its March 2003 meeting that only three of the participating HMOs have funding to collect data on adults. For the vaccines routinely administered to older adults, primarily the influenza and pneumococcal vaccines, Medicare databases may prove to be useful resources for exploratory analyses. A new project to use Medicare data for this purpose was described at that meeting (Burwen, 2003). **The committee recommends efforts to develop techniques for the detection and evaluation of rare adverse events and encourages the use of administrative databases and the standardization of immunization records as part of this effort.**

Basic and Clinical Sciences

Despite advances over the past 25 years in the broad understanding of the pathogenesis of autoimmune diseases and of GBS in particular, the exact mechanisms by which the 1976 influenza vaccines precipitated this adverse outcome remain unknown. To gain a better understanding of these mechanisms, the committee sees a need for additional basic and clinical research on influenza viruses, the composition and immunological properties of the 1976 vaccine, immunological responses to vaccines in general, and host characteristics that may affect susceptibility to adverse events.

There is a need to better understand the immunological responses in recipients of the 1976 swine influenza vaccine who experienced GBS. One avenue of inquiry should be the pathogenesis of influenza viruses in general and the swine influenza strain (A/New Jersey/76) in particular to learn whether and how strains might differ in their ability or predisposition to produce neurological injury. **The committee supports ongoing research aimed at better understanding the pathogenesis of influenza and encourages efforts to anticipate which strains might be more neurologically active.**

Although, the 1976 influenza vaccines were produced under atypical conditions, with the four manufacturers given less time than usual while being asked to produce much larger quantities than in previous years, there is no evidence that the speed of manufacture or volume of production produced lapses that could have led to a faulty vaccine. Even though the viral strain was first identified less than 8 months before vaccination began, about 150 million doses of vaccine were ultimately manufactured (Dowdle, 1997). The increased risk of GBS associated with the 1976 swine influenza vaccines appeared consistent for vaccine from the four different manufacturers, for the monovalent and bivalent vaccines, and for the whole- and split-virus vaccines. The consistency of the risk across the sources and types of vaccine argues against, but does not rule out, problems related to the manufacturing process. Issues that might be investigated include whether there was something atypical about the nonviral components of the swine influenza vaccines and, if so, identifying it and determining whether it can be controlled.

The use of eggs to produce vaccine-strain influenza virus suggests the possibility that unrecognized antigens might have been present in the 1976 vaccine. *C. jejuni* infection is a recognized risk factor for GBS, possibly acting through molecular mimicry, and *C. jejuni* commonly infects chickens. Although the committee concluded that molecular mimicry is only theoretically possible as an immune mechanism by which influenza vaccines may cause GBS, the evidence that *C. jejuni* antigens can trigger GBS is strong, and the possibility cannot be excluded that *C. jejuni* antigens were present in swine influenza vaccines from all four manufacturers of the 1976 swine influenza vaccines. **Although stocks of the 1976 vaccine are unlikely available, the committee recommends that if samples of the influenza vaccines used in 1976 are available, they should be** analyzed for the presence of *C. jejuni* antigens, NS1 or NS2 proteins, or other possible contaminants. The 1976 vaccines should be compared with current and other historical influenza vaccines.

Studies in animals (Hjorth et al., 1984; Ziegler et al., 1983) have provided at least some basis for considering bystander activation as a potential mechanism by which influenza vaccines could cause GBS or related neurological complications. Under contrived experimental conditions, influenza vaccines had adjuvant properties in the presence of neural antigens. But whether an immune system mechanism of this sort played any role in vaccine-related cases of GBS remains far from clear. As it did in a previous report (IOM, 2002a), **the committee recommends continued research using animal and *in vitro* models, as well as with humans, on the mechanisms of immune-mediated neurological diseases that might be associated with exposure to vaccines.**

Genetic factors are known to be an important source of variability in the responses of the human immune system and in the risks of autoimmune disease. The encephalitis/encephalopathy observed as a complication of influenza illness in Japanese children, but only very rarely reported in the United States, suggests the possibility that a genetic factor may be involved in neurological complications of influenza illness. Indications of selective susceptibility to GBS following infection with *C. jejuni* also appear to point to differences in genetic or other host factors, some of which might be relevant as well to examination of mechanisms of vaccine-related risk in 1976 or other years. At present, understanding of the complex interactions among genetic variables and environmental exposures, including vaccines and wild-type infectious organisms, remains incomplete. **The committee recommends continued research efforts aimed at identifying genetic variability in human immune system responsiveness as a way to gain a better understanding of genetic susceptibility to vaccine-based adverse events.**

Communication

It is important that modifications to influenza communication not be seen as independent activities; it is essential that revisions be integrated in an overarching risk management strategy (Bostrom, 1997). While available studies have documented important attitudes, gaps and errors in knowledge, in-depth research is needed to develop greater insights into *why* people have the cognitive limitations, attitudes, and beliefs they have about the influenza vaccine and related issues. This deeper knowledge is necessary to provide an appropriate basis for strengthening risk-benefit communication within an overall risk reduction strategy.

A broader framework for influenza vaccine issues is critical for substantial progress in vaccination rates to be achieved. A rigorous, systematic identification of the influences that affect experts' and subpopulations' views and decisions about vaccines is an important step toward developing such a framework (Bostrom, 1997). Despite the studies that have been conducted to date, a comprehensive context has not yet been compiled for the influenza vaccine. **The committee recommends that research be supported to conduct investigations that would deepen and expand the knowledge available from existing studies and more effectively organize what is currently known from these and future projects.** Comprehensive influence diagrams of expert and at-risk populations' views of the vaccine are needed to provide a broader context and reveal richer insights than are possible from a review of currently available studies.

SUMMARY

Infection with the influenza virus can have a serious effect on the health of people of all ages, although it is particularly worrisome for infants, the elderly, and people with underlying heart or lung problems. At least 35,000 people die in the United States every year from influenza infection. A vaccine exists (the "flu" shot) that can greatly decrease the impact of influenza. Because the strains of virus that are expected to cause serious illness and death are slightly different every year, the vaccine is also slightly different every year and it must be given every year, unlike other vaccines. The influenza vaccine that was used in 1976 for the expected "Swine Flu" epidemic (which never materialized) was associated with cases of a nervous system condition called Guillain-Barré syndrome (GBS). Ever since that time, public health leaders, doctors and nurses, and the public have wondered whether every year's influenza vaccine can cause GBS or other similar conditions.

The Immunization Safety Review committee reviewed the data on influenza vaccine and neurological conditions and concluded that the evidence favored acceptance of a causal relationship between the 1976 swine influenza vaccine and GBS in adults. The evidence about GBS for other years' influenza vaccines is not clear one way or the other (that is, the evidence is inadequate to accept or reject a causal relationship).

The committee concluded that the evidence favored rejection of a causal relationship between influenza vaccines and exacerbation of multiple sclerosis. For the other neurological conditions studied, the committee concluded the evidence about the effects of influenza vaccine is inadequate to accept or reject a causal relationship. The committee also reviewed theories on how the influenza vaccine could damage the nervous system. The evidence was at most weak that the vaccine could act in humans in ways that could lead to these neurological problems. See Box 4 for a summary of all conclusions and recommendations.

BOX 4
Committee Conclusions and Recommendations

SCIENTIFIC ASSESSMENT
Causality Conclusions

The committee concludes that the evidence favors acceptance of a causal relationship between 1976 swine influenza vaccine and Guillain-Barré syndrome in adults.

The committee concludes that the evidence is inadequate to accept or reject a causal relationship between GBS in adults and influenza vaccines administered after 1976 (that is, subsequent to the swine influenza vaccine program).

The committee concludes that the evidence favors rejection of a causal relationship between influenza vaccines and relapse of multiple sclerosis in adults.

The committee concludes that the evidence is inadequate to accept or reject a causal relationship between influenza vaccines and incident MS in adults.

The committee concludes that the evidence is inadequate to accept or reject a causal relationship between influenza vaccines and optic neuritis in adults.

The committee concludes that the evidence is inadequate to accept or reject a causal relationship between influenza vaccines and other demyelinating neurological disorders.

The committee concludes that there is no evidence bearing on a causal relationship between influenza vaccines and demyelinating neurological disorders in children aged 6-23 months.

Biological Mechanisms Conclusions

The committee concludes that there is weak evidence for biological mechanisms related to immune-mediated processes, including molecular mimicry and bystander activation, by which receipt of any influenza vaccine could possibly influence an individual's risk of developing the neurological complications of GBS, MS, or other demyelinating conditions such as optic neuritis.

In the absence of experimental or human evidence regarding the direct neurotoxic effect of influenza vaccines, the committee concludes that this mechanism is only theoretical.

continues

BOX 4 continued

PUBLIC HEALTH RESPONSE RECOMMENDATIONS
Policy Review

The committee does not recommend a policy review of the recommendations for influenza vaccination by any of the national or federal vaccine advisory bodies on the basis of concerns about neurological complications. Current and future immunization policies should continue to reflect the benefits of influenza vaccination.

Research

The committee recommends increased surveillance of adverse events associated with influenza vaccination of children, with particular attentiveness to detecting and assessing potential neurological complications. Enhanced surveillance should be in place before an ACIP recommendation is implemented for universal annual influenza vaccination of young children.

The committee recommends efforts to develop techniques for the detection and evaluation of rare adverse events and encourages the use of administrative databases and the standardization of immunization records as part of this effort.

Basic Science and Clinical Research

The committee supports ongoing research aimed at better understanding the pathogenesis of influenza and encourages efforts to anticipate which strains might be more neurologically active.

Although stocks of the 1976 vaccine are unlikely available, the committee recommends that if samples of the influenza vaccines used in 1976 are available, they should be analyzed for the presence of *C. jejuni* antigens, NS1 or NS2 proteins, or other possible contaminants. The 1976 vaccines should be compared with current and other historical influenza vaccines.

The committee recommends continued research using animal and *in vitro* models, as well as with humans, on the mechanisms of immune-mediated neurological diseases that might be associated with exposure to vaccines.

The committee recommends continued research efforts aimed at identifying genetic variability in human immune system responsiveness as a way to gain a better understanding of genetic susceptibility to vaccine-based adverse events.

Communication

The committee recommends that research be supported to conduct investigations that would deepen and expand the knowledge available from existing studies and more effectively organize what is currently known from these and future projects.

REFERENCES

Albert LJ, Inman RD. 1999. Molecular mimicry and autoimmunity. *N Engl J Med* 341(27):2068–74.

Alter M, Leibowitz U, Speer J. 1966. Risk of multiple sclerosis related to age at immigration to Israel. *Arch Neurol* 15(3):234–7.

Asbury AK. 2000. New concepts of Guillain-Barré syndrome. *J Child Neurol* 15(3):183–91.

ATSDR (Agency for Toxic Substances and Disease Registry). 1999. Toxicological Profile for Mercury (Update).

Bach JF, Chatenoud L. 2001. Tolerance to islet autoantigens in type 1 diabetes. *Annu Rev Immunol* 19:131–61.

Bakshi R, Mazziotta JC. 1996. Acute transverse myelitis after influenza vaccination: magnetic resonance imaging findings. *J Neuroimaging* 6(4):248–50.

Bamford CR, Sibley WA, Laguna JF. 1978. Swine influenza vaccination in patients with multiple sclerosis. *Arch Neurol* 35(4):242–3.

Belshe RB, Couch RB, Glezen WP, Treanor JT. 2002. Live attenuated intranasal influenza vaccine. *Vaccine* 20(29–30):3429–30.

Benoist C, Mathis D. 2001. Autoimmunity provoked by infection: how good is the case for T cell epitope mimicry? *Nat Immunol* 2(9):797–801.

Berna Biotech Ltd. 2002. News Release: Berna Biotech to accelerate development of a 2nd generation nasal flu vaccine product. [online] Available at: http://www.bernabiotech.com/news/archive/article/20020606_01.html [accessed June 6, 2002].

Beyer WE, Palache AM, Osterhaus ADME. 1998. Comparison of serology and reactogenicity between influenza subunit vaccines and whole virus or split vaccines: a review and meta-analysis of the literature. *Clin Drug Invest*; 15(1):1–12.

Beyer WE, Palache AM, de Jong JC, Osterhaus AD. 2002. Cold-adapted live influenza vaccine versus inactivated vaccine: systemic vaccine reactions, local and systemic antibody response, and vaccine efficacy. A meta-analysis. *Vaccine* 20(9-10):1340–53.

Bostrom A. 1997. Vaccine risk communication: Lessons from risk perception, decision making and environmental risk communication research. *Risk*. [online] Available at: http://www.piercelaw.edu/risk/vol8/spring/bostrom.htm.

Breman JG, Hayner NS. 1984. Guillain-Barré syndrome and its relationship to swine influenza vaccination in Michigan, 1976-1977. *Am J Epidemiol* 119(6):880–9.

Bridges C, Thompson W, Meltzer M, Reeve G, Talamonti W, Cox N, Lilac H, Hall H, Klimov A, Fukuda K. 2000. Effectiveness and cost-benefit of influenza vaccination of healthy working adults: a randomized controlled trial. *JAMA* 284(13):1655–63.

Brooks R, Reznik A. 1980. Guillain-Barré syndrome following trivalent influenza vaccine in an elderly patient. *Mt Sinai J Med* 47(2):190–1.

Brostoff SW, White TM. 1982. Absence of P2 protein in swine flu vaccines. *JAMA* 247(4):495.

Burwen D. 2003 (March 13). *Use of Medicare Data to Evaluate Adverse Events After Influenza Vaccine*. Presentation to the Institute of Medicine Meeting on Influenza Vaccine and Neurological Complications, Washington, DC. Institute of Medicine. Immunization Safety Review Committee.

Buzby JC, Allos BM, Roberts T. 1997. The economic burden of *Campylobacter*-associated Guillain-Barré syndrome. *J Infect Dis* 176 Suppl 2:S192–7.

CDC.1999. Primary and Secondary Syphilis—United States, 1998. *MMWR* 48(30):885–90.

CDC. 2002a. *Epidemiology and Prevention of Vaccine-Preventable Diseases 7th Edition*. Public Health Foundation.

CDC. 2002b. Prevention and Control of Influenza: recommendations of the Advisory Committee on Immunization Practices (ACIP); *MMWR Morb Mortal Wkly Rep* 51(RR03):1–31.

CDC. 2002c. Surveillance for Influenza—United States, 1997–98, 1998–99, and 1999–00 Seasons. *MMWR Morb Mortal Wkly Rep* 51(SS-7):1–10.

CDC. 2003a. Infant Botulism— New York City, 2001-2002. *MMWR Morb Mortal Wkly Rep* 52 (2):26–28.

CDC. 2003b. Influenza and Pneumococcal Immunization: a Qualitative Assessment of the Beliefs of Physicians and Older Hispanic and African Americans. [online] Available at: http://www.cdc.gov/nip/flu/flu_qualresearch.htm. [accessed September 9, 2003].

CDC. 2003c. National Center for Infectious Diseases. *Influenza: The Disease.* [online] Available at: www.cdc.gov/ncidod/diseases/flu/fluinfo.htm [accessed March 20, 2003].

CDC. 2003d. Prevention and control of influenza: Recomendations of the Advisory Committee on Immunization Practices (ACIP). *MMWR Morb Mortal Wkly Rep* 52 (RR08):1–36.

CDC. 2003e. Personal Communication with P. Haber. VAERS reports. March, 2003.

Cha TA, Kao K, Zhao J, Fast PE, Mendelman PM, Arvin A. 2000. Genotypic stability of cold-adapted influenza virus vaccine in an efficacy clinical trial. *J Clin Microbiol* 38(2):839–45.

Chen R. 2003 (March 13). *Studies Of Guillain-Barré Syndrome (GBS) After Influenza Vaccination.* Presentation to the Immunization Safety Review Committee, Washington, DC.

Confavreux C, Suissa S, Saddier P, Bourdes V, Vukusic S, for the Vaccines in Multiple Sclerosis Study Group. 2001. Vaccinations and the risk of relapse in multiple sclerosis. *N Engl J Med* 344(5):319–326.

Davidson A, Diamond B. 2001. Autoimmune diseases. *N Engl J Med* 345(5):340–50.

De Keyser J, Zwanikken C, Boon M. 1998. Effects of influenza vaccination and influenza illness on exacerbations in multiple sclerosis. *J Neurol Sci* 159(1):51–3.

Department of Health and Human Services (DHHS). 2003. Product Approval Information. [online] Available at: www.fda.gov/cber/approvltr/inflmed061703L.htm [accessed July 16, 2003].

DeStefano F, Verstraeten T, Jackson LA, Okoro C, Benson P, Black S, Shinefield H, Mullooly P, Likosky W, Chen R. 2003. Vaccinations and risk of central nervous system demyelinating diseases in adults. *Arch Neurol* 60:504–9.

Dolin R. 2001. Influenza. In: Braunwald E, Fauci AS, Kasper DL, Hauser SL, Longo DL, Jameson JL, eds. *Harrison's Principles of Internal Medicine.* 15th ed. New York: McGraw-Hill. Pp. 1125–30.

Dowdle WR. 1997. Pandemic influenza: confronting a re-emergent threat. The 1976 experience. *J Infect Dis* 176 Suppl 1:S69–72.

Ellenberg S, Chen R. 1997. The complicated task of monitoring vaccine safety. *Public Health Reports* 112:10–20.

EPA (Environmental Protection Agency). 1997. *Mercury Study Report to Congress: Volume 1 Executive Summary.* EPA 452/R-97-003.

Evans DM, Dunn G, Minor PD, Schild GC, Cann AJ, Stanway G, Almond JW, Currey K, Maizel JV. 1985. Nature 11-17;314(6011):548–50

Fischoff B, Slovic P, Lichtenstein S, Read S, Combs B. 2000. How safe is safe enough? A psychometric study of attitudes toward technological risks and benefits. In: Slovic P, ed. *The Perception of Risk.* London: Earthscan Publications.

France E. 2003 (March 13). *Safety of the Trivalent Inactivated Influenza Vaccine (TIV) Among Children: A Population-Based Study.* Presentation to the Immunization Safety Review Committee. Washington, DC.

Fu TM, Guan L, Friedman A, Schofield TL, Ulmer JB, Liu MA, Donnelly JJ. 1999. Dose dependence of CTL precursor frequency induced by a DNA vaccine and correlation with protective immunity against influenza virus challenge. *J Immunol* 162(7):4163–70.

Geier M, Geier D, Zahalsky A. 2003. Influenza vaccination and Guillain-Barré syndrome. *Clin Immun* 107 (2003):116–21.

Gonzalez M, Pirez MC, Ward E, Dibarboure H, Garcia A, Picolet H. 2000. Safety and immunogenicity of a paediatric presentation of an influenza vaccine. *Arch Dis Child* 83(6):488–91.

Griffin J. 2003 (March 13). *Guillain-Barré Syndrome.* Presentation to the Immunization Safety Review Committee. Washington, DC..

Haber P. 2003 (March 13). *Influenza Vaccine and Neurological Adverse Events. VAERS 7/1990 - 1/ 2003.* Presentation to the Immunization Safety Review Committee. Washington, DC.

Hahn AF. 1996. Experimental allergic neuritis (EAN) as a model for the immune-mediated demyelinating neuropathies. *Rev Neurol (Paris)* 152(5):328–32.

Halperin SA, Smith B, Mabrouk T, Germain M, Trepanier P, Hassell T, Treanor J, Gauthier R, Mills EL. 2002. Safety and immunogenicity of a trivalent, inactivated, mammalian cell culture-derived influenza vaccine in healthy adults, seniors, and children. *Vaccine* 20(7-8):1240–7.

Hamada T, Driscoll BF, Kies MW, Alvord EC Jr. 1989. LPS augments adoptive transfer of experimental allergic encephalomyelitis in the Lewis rat. *Autoimmunity* 2(4):275–84.

Hilleman MR. 2002. Realities and enigmas of human viral influenza: pathogenesis, epidemiology and control. *Vaccine* 20(25-26):3068–87.

Hjorth RN, Bonde GM, Piner E, Hartzell RW, Rorke LB, Rubin BA. 1984. Experimental neuritis induced by a mixture of neural antigens and influenza vaccines. A possible model for Guillain-Barré syndrome. *J Neuroimmunol* 6(1):1–8.

Hochberg F, Nelson K, Janzen W. 1975. Influenza type B-related encephalopathy. The 1971 outbreak of Reye syndrome in Chicago. *JAMA* 231(8):817–21.

Houff SA, Miller GL, Lovell CR, Wallen WC, Madden DL, Sever JL, Dolin R. 1977. The Guillain-Barré syndrome and swine influenza vaccination. *Trans Am Neurol Assoc* 102:120–3.

Hughes RA, Rees JH. 1997. Clinical and epidemiologic features of Guillain-Barré syndrome. *J Infect Dis* 176 Suppl 2:S92–8.

Hughes RA, Raphael JC, Swan AV, van Doorn PA. 2001. Intravenous immunoglobulin for Guillain-Barré syndrome. *Cochrane Database Syst Rev* (2):CD002063.

Hurwitz ES, Schonberger LB, Nelson DB, Holman RC. 1981. Guillain-Barré syndrome and the 1978–1979 influenza vaccine. *N Engl J Med* 304(26):1557–61.

IOM (Institute of Medicine). 1991. *Adverse Events Following Pertussis and Rubella Vaccines.* Washington DC: National Academy Press.

IOM (Institute of Medicine).1994a. *Adverse Events Associated with Childhood Vaccines: Evidence Bearing on Causality.* Washington DC: National Academy Press.

IOM (Institute of Medicine). 1994b. *DPT Vaccine and Chronic Nervous System Dysfunction: A New Analysis.* Washington DC: National Academy Press.

IOM (Institute of Medicine). 2001a. *Immunization Safety Review: Measles-Mumps-Rubella Vaccine and Autism.* Washington, DC: National Academy Press.

IOM (Institute of Medicine). 2001b. *Immunization Safety Review: Thimerosal-Containing Vaccines and Neurodevelopmental Disorders.* Washington DC: National Academy Press.

IOM (Institute of Medicine). 2001c. *Multiple Sclerosis: Current Status and Strategies for the Future.* Washington DC: National Academy Press.

IOM (Institute of Medicine). 2002a. *Immunization Safety Review: Hepatitis B Vaccine and Demyelinating Neurological Disorders.* Washington DC: National Academy Press.

IOM (Institute of Medicine). 2002b. *Immunization Safety Review: Multiple Immunizations and Immune Dysfunction.* Washington DC: National Academy Press.

IOM (Institute of Medicine). 2002c. *Immunization Safety Review: SV40 Contamination of Polio Vaccine and Cancer.* Washington, DC: The National Academies Press.

IOM (Institute of Medicine). 2003. *Immunization Safety Review: Sudden Uxexpected Death in Infancy.* Washington, DC: The National Academies Press.

Jacobs BC, Rothbarth PH, van der Meche FG, Herbrink P, Schmitz PI, de Klerk MA, van Doorn PA. 1998. The spectrum of antecedent infections in Guillain-Barré syndrome: a case-control study. *Neurology* 51(4):1110–5.

Jahnke U, Fischer EH, Alvord EC Jr. 1985. Sequence homology between certain viral proteins and proteins related to encephalomyelitis and neuritis. *Science* 229(4710):282–4.

Johnson DE. 1982. Guillain-Barré syndrome in the U.S. Army. *Arch Neurol* 39(1):21–4.

Joseph SA, Tsao CY. 2002. Guillain-Barré syndrome. *Adolesc Med* 13(3):487–94.

Kaplan JE, Katona P, Hurwitz ES, Schonberger LB. 1982. Guillain-Barré syndrome in the United States, 1979–1980 and 1980-1981. Lack of an association with influenza vaccination. *JAMA* 248(6):698–700.

Kawasaki A, Purvin VA, Tang R. 1998. Bilateral anterior ischemic optic neuropathy following influenza vaccination. *J Neuroophthalmol* 18(1):56–9.

Keegan BM, Noseworthy JH. 2002. Multiple sclerosis. *Annu Rev Med* 53:285–302.

Keenlyside RA, Schonberger LB, Bregman DJ, Bolyai JZ. 1980. Fatal Guillain-Barré syndrome after the national influenza immunization program. *Neurology* 30(9):929–33.

Kilbourne ED, Arden NH. 1999. Inactivated Influenza. In: Plotkin SA, Orenstein W, eds. *Vaccines.* 3rd ed. Philadelphia: W.B. Saunders Company. Pp. 531–51.

Kinnunen E, Junttila O, Haukka J, Hovi T. 1998. Nationwide oral poliovirus vaccination campaign and the incidence of Guillain-Barré syndrome. *Am J Epidemiol* 147(1):69–73.

Kitch EW, Evans G, Gobin R. 1999. U.S. law. In: Plotkin SA, Orenstein W, eds. *Vaccines.* 3rd ed. Philadelphia: W.B. Saunders Company.Pp. 1165–67.

Knight RS, Duncan JS, Davis CJ, Warlow CP. 1984. Influenza vaccination and Guillain-Barré syndrome. *Lancet* 1(8373):394.

Kurland LT, Molgaard CA, Kurland EM, Wiederholt WC, Kirkpatrick JW. 1984. Swine flu vaccine and multiple sclerosis. *JAMA* 251(20):2672–5.

Kurland LT, Wiederholt WC, Beghe E, Kirkpatrick JW, Potter HG, Armstrong FP. 1986. Guillain-Barré syndrome following (a/New Jersey/76) influenza (swine flu) vaccine: epidemic or artifact? In Poeck K, Freund HJ, Gänshirt H, eds. *Neurology: Proceedings of the XIIIth World Congress of Neurology, Hamburg, September 1-6, 1985.* Berlin; New York: Springer-Verlag.

Kurtzke JF, Beebe GW, Nagler B, Nefzger MD, Auth TL, Kurland LT. 1970. Studies on the natural history of multiple sclerosis. V. Long-term survival in young men. *Arch Neurol* 22(3):215–25.

Langmuir AD. 1979. Guillain-Barré syndrome: the swine influenza virus vaccine incident in the United States of America, 1976–77: preliminary communication. *J R Soc Med* 72(9):660–9.

Langmuir AD, Bregman DJ, Kurland LT, Nathanson N, Victor M. 1984. An epidemiologic and clinical evaluation of Guillain-Barré syndrome reported in association with the administration of swine influenza vaccines. *Am J Epidemiol* 119(6):841–79.

Larner AJ, Farmer SF. 2000. Myelopathy following influenza vaccination in inflammatory CNS disorder treated with chronic immunosuppression. *Eur J Neurol* 7(6):731–3.

Lasky T. 2003 (March 13). *Influenza Vaccine and GBS.* Presentation to the Immunization Safety Review Commitee. Washington, DC.

Lasky T, Terracciano GJ, Magder L, Koski CL, Ballesteros M, Nash D, Clark S, Haber P, Stolley PD, Schonberger LB, Chen RT. 1998. The Guillain-Barré syndrome and the 1992–1993 and 1993–1994 influenza vaccines. *N Engl J Med* 339(25):1797–802.

Leask JA, Chapman S. 1998. An attempt to swindle nature: press anti-immunization reportage 1993–1997. *Aust N Z J Public Health* 22(1):17–26.

Ledeen R. 1985. Gangliosides of the neuron. *Trends Neurosci* 8(4):169–174.

Levandowski R. 2003 (March 13). *Influenza Vaccine Production.* Presentation to the Immunization Safety Review Committee. Washington, DC.

Lin YP, Shaw M, Gregory V, Cameron K, Lim W, Klimov A, Subbarao K, Guan Y, Krauss S, Shortridge K, Webster R, Cox N, Hay A. 2000. Avian-to-human transmission of H9N2 subtype influenza A viruses: relationship between H9N2 and H5N1 human isolates. *Proc Natl Acad Sci U S A* 97(17):9654–8.

Lublin FD, Reingold SC. 1996. Defining the clinical course of multiple sclerosis: results of an international survey. National Multiple Sclerosis Society (USA) Advisory Committee on Clinical Trials of New Agents in Multiple Sclerosis. *Neurology* 46(4):907–11.

Maassab HF, Bryant ML. 1999. The development of live attenuated cold-adapted influenza virus vaccine for humans. *Rev Med Virol* 9(4):237–44.

Magira EE, Papaioakim M, Nachamkin I, Asbury AK, Li CY, Ho TW, Griffin JW, McKhann GM, Monos DS. 2003. Differential distribution of HLA-DQ beta/DR beta epitopes in the two forms of Guillain-Barré syndrome, acute motor axonal neuropathy and acute inflammatory demyelinating polyneuropathy (AIDP): identification of DQ beta epitopes associated with susceptibility to and protection from AIDP. *J Immunol* 170(6):3074–80.

Marks JS, Halpin TJ. 1980. Guillain-Barré syndrome in recipients of A/New Jersey influenza vaccine. *JAMA* 243(24):2490–4.

Marrack P, Kappler J, Kotzin BL. 2001. Autoimmune disease: why and where it occurs. *Nat Med* 7(8):899–905.

Miller AE, Morgante LA, Buchwald LY, Nutile SM, Coyle PK, Krupp LB, Doscher CA, Lublin FD, Knobler RL, Trantas F, Kelley L, Smith CR, La Rocca N, Lopez S. 1997. A multicenter, randomized, double-blind, placebo-controlled trial of influenza immunization in multiple sclerosis. *Neurology* 48(2):312–4.

Mokhtarian F, Shirazian D, Morgante L, Miller A, Grob D, Lichstein E. 1997. Influenza virus vaccination of patients with multiple sclerosis. *Mult Scler* 3(4):243–7.

Moran AP, Prendergast MM. 2001. Molecular mimicry in *Campylobacter jejuni* and *Helicobacter pylori* lipopolysaccharides: contribution of gastrointestinal infections to autoimmunity. *J Autoimmun* 16(3):241–56.

Moran AP, Prendergast MM, Hogan EL. 2002. Sialosyl-galactose: a common denominator of Guillain-Barré and related disorders. *J Neurol Sci* 196(1-2):1–7.

Morishima T, Togashi T, Yokota S, Okuno Y, Miyazaki C, Tashiro M, Okabe N. 2002. Encephalitis and encephalopathy associated with an influenza epidemic in Japan. *Clin Infect Dis* 35(5):512–7.

Myers LW, Ellison GW, Lucia M, Novom S, Holevoet M, Madden D, Sever J, Noble GR. 1977. Swine influenza virus vaccination in patients with multiple sclerosis. *J Infect Dis* 136 Suppl:S546–54.

Nachamkin I. 2002. Rabbit model of Guillain-Barré syndrome. *Ann Neurol* 52(1):127–8.

National Institute of Neurological Disorders and Stroke (NINDS). 2001. Guillain-Barré Syndrome Information Page. [Online]. Available: http://www.ninds.nih.gov/health_and_medical/disorders/gbs.htm [accessed March 20, 2003].

Neirynck S, Deroo T, Saelens X, Vanlandschoot P, Jou WM, Fiers W. 1999. A universal influenza A vaccine based on the extracellular domain of the M2 protein. *Nat Med* 5(10):1157–63.

Neuzil KM, Dupont WD, Wright PF, Edwards KM. 2001. Efficacy of inactivated and cold-adapted vaccines against influenza A infection, 1985 to 1990: the pediatric experience. *Pediatr Infect Dis J* 20(8):733–40.

Newland JG, Romero JR, Varman M, Drake C, Holst A, Safranek T, Subbarao K. 2003. Encephalitis associated with influenza B virus infection in 2 children and a review of the literature. *Clin Infect Dis* 36(7):87–95.

Nichol K. 2001. Cost-benefit analysis of a strategy to vaccinate healthy working adults against influenza. *Arch Intern Med* 161(5):749–59.

Noseworthy JH, Lucchinetti C, Rodriguez M, Weinshenker BG. 2000. Multiple sclerosis. *N Engl J Med* 343(13):938–52.

NRC (National Research Council). 2000. *Toxicological Effects of Methylmercury.* Washington, D.C.: National Academy Press.

Okuda K, Ihata A, Watabe S, Okada E, Yamakawa T, Hamajima K, Yang J, Ishii N, Nakazawa M, Okuda K, Ohnari K, Nakajima K, Xin KQ. 2001. Protective immunity against influenza A virus induced by immunization with DNA plasmid containing influenza M gene. *Vaccine* 19(27):3681–91.

Osler LD, Sidell AD. 1960. The Guillain-Barré syndrome. *N Engl J Med* 262:964–969.

Palese P, Garcia-Sastre A. 2002. Influenza vaccines: present and future. *J Clin Invest* 110(1):9–13.

Parkin WE, Beecham HJ, Streiff E, Sharrar RG, Harris JC. 1978. Relationship studied in Pennsylvania. Guillain-Barré syndrome and influenza immunization. *Pa Med* 81(4):47–8, 50–2.

PDR. 2003. Physicians Desk Reference, 57th edition. Thomson PDR. Montvale, NJ.

Pfleiderer M, Lower J, Kurth R. 2001. Cold-attenuated live influenza vaccines, a risk-benefit assessment. *Vaccine* 20(5-6):886–94.

Piedra PA, Glezen WP, Mbawuike I, Gruber WC, Baxter BD, Boland FJ, Byrd RW, Fan LL, Lewis JK, Rhodes LJ, Whitney SE, Taber LH. 1993. Studies on reactogenicity and immunogenicity of attenuated bivalent cold recombinant influenza type A (CRA) and inactivated trivalent influenza virus (TI) vaccines in infants and young children. *Vaccine* 11(7):718–24.

Plotkin SA, Rupprecht CE, Koprowski H. 1995. Rabies vaccine. In: Plotkin SA, Orenstein W, eds. *Vaccines*. 3rd ed. Philadelphia: W.B. Saunders Company. Pp. 743–66.

Poser CM, Behan PO. 1982. Late onset of Guillain-Barré syndrome. *J Neuroimmunol* 3(1):27–41.

Poser CM, Roman G, Emery ES. 1978. Recurrent disseminated vasculomyelinopathy. *Arch Neurol* 35(3):166–70.

Poser CM, Paty DW, Scheinberg L, McDonald WI, Davis FA, Ebers GC, Johnson KP, Sibley WA, Silberberg DH, Tourtellotte WW. 1983. New diagnostic criteria for multiple sclerosis: guidelines for research protocols. *Ann Neurol* 13(3):227–31.

Postic B, Delaney JF, Miller RA. 1980. Landry-Guillain-Barré syndrome following influenza A/New Jersey/76 vaccine: case report. *Mil Med* 145(8):561–2.

Purvin V. 1998. Optic neuritis. *Curr Opin Ophthalmol* 9(6):3–9.

Rantala H, Cherry JD, Shields WD, Uhari M. 1994. Epidemiology of Guillain-Barré syndrome in children: relationship of oral polio vaccine administration to occurrence. *J Pediatr* 124(2):220–3.

Raphael JC, Chevret S, Hughes RA, Annane D. 2001. Plasma exchange for Guillain-Barré syndrome. *Cochrane Database Syst Rev* (2):CD001798.

Ray CL, Dreizin IJ. 1996. Bilateral optic neuropathy associated with influenza vaccination. *J Neuroophthalmol* 16(3):182–4.

Regner M, Lambert PH. 2001. Autoimmunity through infection or immunization? *Nat Immunol* 2(3):185–8.

Retailliau HF, Curtis AC, Storr G, Caesar G, Eddins DL, Hattwick MA. 1980. Illness after influenza vaccination reported through a nationwide surveillance system, 1976–1977. *Am J Epidemiol* 111(3):270–8.

Roscelli JD, Bass JW, Pang L. 1991. Guillain-Barré syndrome and influenza vaccination in the U.S. Army, 1980–1988. *Am J Epidemiol* 133(9):952–5.

Rose NR. 2001. Infection, mimics, and autoimmune disease. *J Clin Invest* 107(8):943–4.

Safranek TJ, Lawrence DN, Kurland LT, Culver DH, Wiederholt WC, Hayner NS, Osterholm MT, O'Brien P, Hughes JM. 1991. Reassessment of the association between Guillain-Barré syndrome and receipt of swine influenza vaccine in 1976–1977: results of a two-state study. Expert Neurology Group. *Am J Epidemiol* 133(9):940–51.

Saito H, Endo M, Takase S, Itahara K. 1980. Acute disseminated encephalomyelitis after influenza vaccination. *Arch Neurol* 37(9):564–6.

Salvetti M, Pisani A, Bastianello S, Millefiorini E, Buttinelli C, Pozzilli C. 1995. Clinical and MRI assessment of disease activity in patients with multiple sclerosis after influenza vaccination. *J Neurol* 242(3):143–6.

Salvetti M, Pisani A, Bastianello S, Millefiorini E, Buttinelli C, Pozzilli C. 1997. Influenza immunization in multiple sclerosis. *Neurology* 49(5):1474–5.

Schonberger LB, Bregman DJ, Sullivan-Bolyai JZ, Keenlyside RA, Ziegler DW, Retailliau HF, Eddins DL, Bryan JA. 1979. Guillain-Barré syndrome following vaccination in the National Influenza Immunization Program, United States, 1976-1977. *Am J Epidemiol* 110(2):105–23.

Seyal M, Ziegler DK, Couch JR. 1978. Recurrent Guillain-Barré syndrome following influenza vaccine. *Neurology* 28(7):725–6.

Shaw SY, Laursen RA, Lees MB. 1986. Analogous amino acid sequences in myelin proteolipid and viral proteins. *FEBS Lett* 207(2):266–70.

Sheikh KA, Ho TW, Nachamkin I, Li CY, Cornblath DR, Asbury AK, Griffin JW, McKhann GM. 1998. Molecular mimicry in Guillain-Barré syndrome. *Ann N Y Acad Sci* 845:307–21.

Sheremata W, Eylar EH, Szymanska I, Sazant A. 1981. Peripheral nerve myelin P2 protein in influenza vaccine. *Trans Am Neurol Assoc* 106:221–3.

Sibley WA, Bamford CR, Laguna JF. 1976. Influenza vaccination in patients with multiple sclerosis. *JAMA* 236(17):1965–6.

Simonsen L, Fukuda K, Schonberger LB, Cox NJ. 2000. The impact of influenza epidemics on hospitalizations. *J Infect Dis* 181(3):831–7.

Singh B. 2000. Stimulation of the developing immune system can prevent autoimmunity. *J Autoimmun* 14(1):15–22.

Singleton JA, Lloyd JC, Mootrey GT, Salive ME, Chen RT. 1999. An overview of the vaccine adverse event reporting system (VAERS) as a surveillance system. *Vaccine* 17:2908–17.

Steinhauer DA, Skehel JJ. 2002. Genetics of influenza viruses. *Annu Rev Genet* 36:305–32.

Stuve O, Zamvil SS. 1999. Pathogenesis, diagnosis, and treatment of acute disseminated encephalomyelitis. *Curr Opin Neurol* 12(4):395–401.

Sugaya N. 2002. Influenza-associated encephalopathy in Japan. *Semin Pediatr Infect Dis* 13(2):79-84.

Sunderrajan EV, Davenport J. 1985. The Guillain-Barré syndrome: pulmonary-neurologic correlations. *Medicine* 64(5):333–41.

Sutter RW, Cochi SL, Melnick JL. 1999. Live attenuated poliovirus vaccines. In: Plotkin SA, Orenstein W, eds. *Vaccines.* 3rd ed. Philadelphia: W.B. Saunders Company. Pp. 364–408.

Thompson WW, Shay DK, Weintraub E, Brammer L, Cox N, Anderson LJ, Fukuda K. 2003. Mortality associated with influenza and respiratory syncytial virus in the United States. *JAMA* 289(2):179–86.

Vriesendorp FJ. 1997. Insights into *Campylobacter jejuni*-induced Guillain-Barré syndrome from the Lewis rat model of experimental allergic neuritis. *J Infect Dis* 176 Suppl 2:S164–8.

Wareing MD, Tannock GA. 2001. Live attenuated vaccines against influenza; an historical review. *Vaccine* 19(25-26):3320–30.

Waubant E, Stuve O. 2002. Suspected mechanisms involved in multiple sclerosis and putative role of hepatitis B vaccine in multiple sclerosis. *Commissioned background paper for IOM Immunization Safety Review Committee.*

Webster RG. 1997. Predictions for future human influenza pandemics. *J Infect Dis* 176 Suppl 1:S14–9.

Webster RG. 1999. 1918 Spanish influenza: the secrets remain elusive. *Proc Natl Acad Sci U S A* 96(4):1164–6.

Webster R. 2003 (March 13). *Influenza.* Presentation to the Immunization Safety Review Committee.Washington, DC. Institute of Medicine.

Weise MJ, Carnegie PR. 1988. An approach to searching protein sequences for superfamily relationships or chance similarities relevant to the molecular mimicry hypothesis: application to the basic proteins of myelin. *J Neurochem* 51(4):1267–73.

Winer JB. 2001. Guillain-Barré syndrome. *Mol Pathol* 54(6):381–5.

Winer JB, Hughes RA, Bradley GW, Scadding JW. 1984. Guillain-Barré syndrome and influenza vaccine. *Lancet* 1(8387):1182.

Wucherpfennig KW. 2001. Mechanisms for the induction of autoimmunity by infectious agents. *J Clin Invest* 108(8):1097–104.

Yahr MD, Lobo-Antunes J. 1972. Relapsing encephalomyelitis following the use of influenza vaccine. *Arch Neurol* 27(2):182–3.

Yoshikawa H, Yamazaki S, Watanabe T, Abe T. 2001. Study of influenza-associated encephalitis/encephalopathy in children during the 1997 to 2001 influenza seasons. *J Child Neurol* 16(12):885–90.

Ziegler DW, Gardner JJ, Warfield DT, Walls HH. 1983. Experimental allergic neuritis-like disease in rabbits after injection with influenza vaccines mixed with gangliosides and adjuvants. *Infect Immun* 42(2):824–30.

Ziegler T, Cox NJ. 1999. Influenza viruses. In: Murray PR, Baron EJ, Pfaller MA, Tenover FC, Yolken, eds. *Manual of Clinical Microbiology.* 7th ed. Washington, DC: ASM Press.

Zimmerman RK, Nowalk MP, Santibanez TA, Jewell IK, Raymond M. 2003a. Shortage of influenza vaccine in 2000-2001: did it change patient beliefs? *Am J Prev Med* 24(4):349–53.

Zimmerman RK, Santibanez TA, Janosky JE, Fine MJ, Raymund M, Wilson SA, Bardella IJ, Medsger AR, Nowalk MP. 2003b. What affects influenza vaccination rates among older patients? An analysis from inner-city, suburban, rural, and Veterans Affairs practices. *Am J Med* 114(1):31–8.

Zinkernagel RM. 2001. Maternal antibodies, childhood infections, and autoimmune diseases. *N Engl J Med* 345(18):1331–5.

Appendix A

Committee Recommendations and Conclusions from Previous Reports

MEASLES-MUMPS-RUBELLA VACCINE AND AUTISM

Conclusions

The committee concludes that the evidence favors rejection of a causal relationship at the population level between measles-mumps-rubella (MMR) vaccine and autistic spectrum disorders (ASD). However, this conclusion does not exclude the possibility that MMR vaccine could contribute to ASD in a small number of children.

The committee concludes that further research on the possible occurrence of ASD in a small number of children subsequent to MMR vaccination is warranted, and it has identified targeted research opportunities that could lead to firmer understanding of the relationship.

Recommendations

Public Health Response

The committee recommends that the relationship between the MMR vaccine and autistic spectrum disorders receive continued attention.

Policy Review

The committee does not recommend a policy review at this time of the licensure of MMR vaccine or of the current schedule and recommendations for administration of MMR vaccine.

Research Regarding MMR and ASD

The committee recommends the use of accepted and consistent case definitions and assessment protocols for ASD in order to enhance the precision and comparability of results from surveillance, epidemiological, and biological investigations.

The committee recommends the exploration of whether exposure to MMR vaccine is a risk factor for autistic spectrum disorder in a small number of children.

The committee recommends the development of targeted investigations of whether or not measles vaccine-strain virus is present in the intestines of some children with ASD.

The committee encourages all who submit reports to VAERS of any diagnosis of ASD thought to be related to MMR vaccine to provide as much detail and as much documentation as possible.

The committee recommends studying the possible effects of different MMR immunization exposures.

The committee recommends conducting further clinical and epidemiological studies of sufficient rigor to identify risk factors and biological markers of ASD in order to better understand genetic or environmental causes.

Communications

The committee recommends that government agencies and professional organizations, CDC and the Food and Drug Administration (FDA) in particular, review some of the most prominent forms of communication regarding the hypothesized relationship between MMR vaccine and ASD, including information they provide via the Internet and the ease with which Internet information can be accessed.

THIMEROSAL-CONTAINING VACCINES AND NEURODEVELOPMENTAL DISORDERS

Conclusions

The committee concludes that although the hypothesis that exposure to thimerosal-containing vaccines could be associated with neurodevelopmental disorders is not established and rests on indirect and incomplete information, primarily from analogies with methylmercury and levels of maximum mercury exposure from vaccines given in children, the hypothesis is biologically plausible.

The committee also concludes that the evidence is inadequate to accept or reject a causal relationship between thimerosal exposures from childhood vaccines and the neurodevelopmental disorders of autism, ADHD, and speech or language delay.

Public Health Response Recommendations

Policy Review and Analysis

The committee recommends the use of the thimerosal-free DTaP, Hib, and hepatitis B vaccines in the United States, despite the fact that there might be remaining supplies of thimerosal-containing vaccine available.

The committee recommends that full consideration be given by appropriate professional societies and government agencies to removing thimerosal from vaccines administered to infants, children, or pregnant women in the United States.

The committee recommends that appropriate professional societies and government agencies review their policies about the non-vaccine biological and pharmaceutical products that contain thimerosal and are used by infants, children, and pregnant women in the United States.

The committee recommends that policy analyses be conducted that will inform these discussions in the future.

The committee recommends a review and assessment of how public health policy decisions are made under uncertainty.

The committee recommends a review of the strategies used to communicate rapid changes in vaccine policy, and it recommends research on how to improve those strategies.

Public Health and Biomedical Research

The committee recommends a diverse public health and biomedical research portfolio.

Epidemiological Research

The committee recommends case-control studies examining the potential link between neurodevelopmental disorders and thimerosal-containing vaccines.

The committee recommends further analysis of neurodevelopmental disorders in cohorts of children who did not receive thimerosal-containing doses as part of a clinical trial of DTaP vaccine.

The committee recommends conducting epidemiological studies that compare the incidence and prevalence of neurodevelopmental disorders before and after the removal of thimerosal from vaccines.

The committee recommends an increased effort to identify the primary sources and levels of prenatal and postnatal background exposure to thimerosal (e.g., Rho (D) Immune Globulin) and other forms of mercury (e.g., maternal consumption of fish) in infants, children, and pregnant women.

Clinical Research

The committee recommends research on how children, including those diagnosed with neurodevelopmental disorders, metabolize and excrete metals—particularly mercury.

The committee recommends continued research on theoretical modeling of ethylmercury exposures, including the incremental burden of thimerosal with background mercury exposure from other sources.

The committee recommends careful, rigorous, and scientific investigations of chelation when used in children with neurodevelopmental disorders, especially autism.

Basic Science Research

The committee recommends research to identify a safe, effective, and inexpensive alternative to thimerosal for countries that decide they need to switch from using thimerosal as a preservative.

The committee recommends research in appropriate animal models on the neurodevelopmental effects of ethylmercury.

MULTIPLE IMMUNIZATIONS AND IMMUNE DYSFUNCTION

Conclusions

Scientific Assessment

Causality Conclusions

The committee concludes that the epidemiological evidence favors rejection of a causal relationship between multiple immunizations and an increase in heterologous infection.

The committee concludes that the epidemiological evidence favors rejection of a causal relationship between multiple immunizations and an increased risk of type 1 diabetes.

The committee concludes that the epidemiological evidence is inadequate to accept or reject a causal relationship between multiple immunizations and increased risk of allergic disease, particularly asthma.

Biological Mechanisms Conclusions

Autoimmune Disease

In the absence of experimental or human evidence regarding molecular mimicry or mercury-induced modification of any vaccine component to create an antigenic epitope capable of cross-reaction with self epitopes as a mechanism by which multiple immunizations under the U.S. infant immunization schedule could possibly influence an individual's risk of autoimmunity, the committee concludes that these mechanisms are only theoretical.

The committee concludes that there is weak evidence for bystander activation, alone or in concert with molecular mimicry, as a mechanism by which multiple immunizations under the U.S. infant immunization schedule could possibly influence an individual's risk of autoimmunity.

In the absence of experimental or human evidence regarding loss of protection against a homologous infection as a mechanism by which multiple immunizations under the U.S. infant immunization schedule could possibly influence an individual's risk of autoimmunity, the committee concludes that this mechanism is only theoretical.

In the absence of experimental or human evidence regarding mechanisms related to the hygiene hypothesis as a means by which multiple immunizations under the U.S. infant immunization schedule could possibly influence an individual's risk of autoimmunity, the committee concludes that this mechanism is only theoretical.

Considering molecular mimicry, bystander activation, and impaired immunoregulation collectively rather than individually, the committee concludes that there is weak evidence for these mechanisms as means by which multiple immunizations under the U.S. infant immunization schedule could possibly influence an individual's risk of autoimmunity.

Allergic Disease

The committee concludes that there is weak evidence for bystander activation as a mechanism by which multiple immunizations under the U.S. infant immunization schedule could possibly influence an individual's risk of allergy.

In the absence of experimental or human evidence regarding mechanisms related to the hygiene hypothesis as a means by which multiple immunizations under the U.S. infant immunization schedule could possibly influence an individual's risk of allergy, the committee concludes that this mechanism is only theoretical.

The committee concludes that there is weak evidence for the existence of any biological mechanisms, collectively or individually, by which multiple immunizations under the U.S. infant immunization schedule could possibly influence an individual's risk of allergy.

Heterologous Infection

The committee concludes that there is strong evidence for the existence of biological mechanisms by which multiple immunizations under the U.S. infant immunization schedule could possibly influence an individual's risk for heterologous infections.

Significance Assessment

The committee concludes that concern about multiple immunizations has been, and could continue to be, of societal significance in terms of parental worries, potential health burdens, and future challenges for immunization policymaking.

Public Health Response Recommendations

Policy Review

The committee recommends that state and federal vaccine policymakers consider a broader and more explicit strategy for developing recommendations for the use of vaccines.

The committee does not recommend a policy review—by the CDC's Advisory Committee on Immunization Practices (ACIP), the American Academy of Pediatrics' Committee on Infectious Diseases, and the American Academy of Family Physicians—of the current recommended childhood immunization schedule on the basis of concerns about immune system dysfunction.

The committee does not recommend a policy review by the Food and Drug Administration's Vaccines and Related Biologic Products Advisory Committee of any currently licensed vaccines on the basis of concerns about immune system dysfunction.

Research

Epidemiological Research

The committee recommends exploring the feasibility of using existing vaccine surveillance systems, alone or in combination, to study safety questions related to asthma and other important allergic disorders, as well as to type 1 diabetes and other important autoimmune diseases.

The committee recommends exploring the use of cohorts for research on possible vaccine-related disease risks. Furthermore, the committee recommends that disease registries and research programs for autoimmune and allergic disorders routinely collect immunization histories as part of their study protocol.

Basic Science and Clinical Research

The committee recommends continued research on the development of the human infant immune system.

The committee endorses current research efforts aimed at identifying genetic variability in human immune system development and immune system responsiveness as a way to gain a better understanding of genetic susceptibility to vaccine-based adverse events.

The committee recommends exploring the feasibility of collecting data on surrogate markers for autoimmune and allergic disorders in the vaccine testing and licensing process.

The committee recommends exploring surrogates for allergy and autoimmunity in existing cohort studies of variations in the vaccine schedule.

Communication

The committee recommends that an appropriate panel of multidisciplinary experts be convened by the Department of Health and Human Services. It would develop a comprehensive research strategy for knowledge leading to the optimal design and evaluation of vaccine risk-benefit communication approaches.

HEPATITIS B VACCINE AND DEMYELINATING NEUROLOGICAL DISORDERS

Scientific Assessment

Causality Conclusions

The committee concludes that the evidence favors rejection of a causal relationship between hepatitis B vaccine administered to adults and incident multiple sclerosis.

The committee also concludes that the evidence favors rejection of a causal relationship between hepatitis B vaccine administered to adults and multiple sclerosis relapse.

The committee concludes that the evidence is inadequate to accept or reject a causal relationship between hepatitis B vaccine and the first episode of a central nervous system demyelinating disorder.

The committee concludes that the evidence is inadequate to accept or reject a causal relationship between hepatitis B vaccine and ADEM.

The committee concludes that the evidence is inadequate to accept or reject a causal relationship between hepatitis B vaccine and optic neuritis.

The committee concludes that the evidence is inadequate to accept or reject a causal relationship between hepatitis B vaccine and transverse myelitis.

The committee concludes that the evidence is inadequate to accept or reject a causal relationship between hepatitis B vaccine and GBS.

The committee concludes that the evidence is inadequate to accept or reject a causal relationship between hepatitis B vaccine and brachial neuritis.

The committee concludes that there is weak evidence for biological mechanisms by which hepatitis B vaccination could possibly influence an individual's risk of the central or peripheral nervous system disorders of MS, first episode of CDD, ADEM, or optic neuritis, transverse myelitis, GBS, or brachial neuritis.

Significance Assessment

The committee concludes that concerns about the hepatitis B vaccine remain significant in the minds of some parents and workers who are required to take the vaccine because of occupational risk.

Public Health Response Recommendations

Policy Review

The committee does not recommend a policy review of the hepatitis B vaccine by any of the national and federal vaccine advisory bodies on the basis of concerns about demyelinating neurological disorders.

The committee recommends continued surveillance of hepatitis B disease and increased surveillance of secondary diseases such as cirrhosis and hepato-cellular carcinoma.

Basic and Clinical Science

The committee recommends continued research in animal and *in vitro* models, as well as in humans, on the mechanisms of immune-mediated neurological disease possibly associated with exposure to vaccines.

Communication

The committee again recommends that government agencies and professional organizations responsible for immunizations critically evaluate their communication services with increased understanding of, and input from, the intended user.

SV40 CONTAMINATION OF POLIO VACCINE AND CANCER

Scientific Assessment

Causality Conclusions

The committee concludes that the evidence is inadequate to accept or reject a causal relationship between SV40-containing polio vaccines and cancer.

Biological Mechanisms Conclusions

The committee concludes that the biological evidence is strong that SV40 is a transforming virus.

The committee concludes that the biological evidence is moderate that SV40 exposure could lead to cancer in humans under natural conditions.

The committee concludes that the biological evidence is moderate that SV40 exposure from the polio vaccine is related to SV40 infection in humans.

Significance Assessment

The committee concludes that concerns about exposure to SV40 through inadvertent contamination of polio vaccines are significant because of the seriousness of cancers as the possible adverse health outcomes and because of the continuing need to ensure and protect public trust in the nation's immunization program.

Public Health Response Recommendations

Policy Review

The committee does not recommend a policy review of polio vaccine by any of the national or federal vaccine advisory bodies, on the basis of concerns about cancer risks that might be associated with exposure to SV40, because the vaccine in current use is free of SV40.

Policy Analysis and Communication

The committee recommends that the appropriate federal agencies develop a Vaccine Contamination Prevention and Response Plan.

Research

The committee recommends development of sensitive and specific serologic tests for SV40.

The committee recommends the development and use of sensitive and specific standardized techniques for SV40 detection.

The committee recommends that once there is agreement in the scientific community as to the best detection methods and protocols, pre-1955 samples of human tissues should be assayed for presence or absence of SV40 in rigorous, multi-center studies.

The committee recommends further study of the transmissibility of SV40 in humans.

Until some of the technical issues are resolved, the committee does not recommend additional epidemiological studies of people potentially exposed to the contaminated polio vaccine.

VACCINATIONS AND SUDDEN UNEXPECTED DEATH IN INFANCY

Scientific Assessment

Causality Conclusions

There is no basis for a change in the prior conclusions that the evidence favors rejection of a causal relationship between DTwP vaccine and SIDS.

The evidence is inadequate to accept or reject a causal relationship between DTaP vaccine and SIDS.

The evidence is inadequate to accept or reject causal relationships between SIDS and the individual vaccines, Hib, HepB, OPV, and IPV.

The evidence favors rejection of a causal relationship between exposure to multiple vaccines and SIDS.

The evidence is inadequate to accept or reject a causal relationship between exposure to multiple vaccines and sudden unexpected death in infancy, other than SIDS.

The evidence favors acceptance of a causal relationship between diphtheria toxoid-and whole cell pertussis vaccine and death due to anaphylaxis in infants.

The evidence is inadequate to accept or reject a causal relationship between hepatitis B vaccine and neonatal death.

Biological Mechanisms Conclusions

In the absence of experimental or human evidence regarding the ability of common side effects of immunization, including fever and anorexia, to trigger sudden unexpected death in infants with underlying neuroregulatory abnormalities, the committee concludes that this mechanisms is only theoretical.

In the absence of experimental or human evidence regarding the ability of common side effects of immunization, including fever and anorexia, to trigger an acute metabolic crisis in patients with inborn errors of metabolism, the committee concludes that this mechanism for vaccine-related sudden unexpected infant death is only theoretical.

In the absence of experimental or human evidence demonstrating the ability of vaccines to stimulate an abnormal inflammatory response in the lung leading to sudden unexpected infant death, the committee concludes that this mechanism is only theoretical.

The committee concludes that immediate type I hypersensitivity reactions to vaccines can cause SUDI within 24 hours of vaccine administration. Although a type I hypersensitivity reaction leading to death could possibly be missed both clinically and at post-mortem examination, and therefore misdiagnosed as SIDS, the committee concludes that this possibility is only theoretical.

Public Health Response Recommendations

Policy Review

The committee does not recommend a policy review of the recommended childhood vaccination schedule by any of the national or federal vaccine advisory bodies on the basis of concerns about sudden unexpected death in infancy.

Surveillance and Epidemiological Studies

The committee urges prompt publication of all Vaccine Safety Datalink results.

Basic and Clinical Science

The committee recommends continued research on the etiology and pathology of SIDS.

The committee recommends that a comprehensive postmortem workup, including a metabolic analysis, be done on all infants who die suddenly and unexpectedly.

The committee encourages efforts by Centers for Disease Control and Prevention, American Academy of Pediatrics, and others to promote the development and consistent use throughout the United States of national guidelines for investigation, diagnosis, and reporting of SIDS cases.

The committee recommends the development of standard definitions and guidance for diagnosis and reporting of SUDI for research purposes.

Appendix B

Public Meeting Agenda
March 13, 2003

Immunization Safety Review
Influenza Vaccine and Possible Neurological Complications

Hotel Monaco
Athens Room, 700 F St., NW
Washington, DC

9:00 – 9:15 am   **Welcome and Opening Remarks**
Marie McCormick, MD, ScD, Committee Chair

9:15 – 9:45 am   **Influenza**
Robert G. Webster, PhD
St. Jude Children's Research Hospital

9:45 – 10:15 am   **Guillain-Barré Syndrome**
John Griffin, MD
The Johns Hopkins University School of Medicine

10:15 – 10:45 am   **The Yearly Production of Influenza Vaccine**
Roland Levandowski, MD
Food and Drug Administration

10:45 – 11:00 am   **Break**

11:00 – 11:30 am	**VAERS Reports Related to Influenza Vaccine** *Penina Haber,MPH* *Centers for Disease Control and Prevention*
11:30 – 12:15 pm	**Discussion**
12:15 – 1:30 pm	**Lunch**
1:30 – 2:15 pm	**Studies of Guillain-Barré Syndrome After Influenza Vaccination** *Robert Chen, MD* *Centers for Disease Control and Prevention*
2:15 – 2:45 pm	**Guillain-Barré Syndrome and the 1992-1993 and 1993-1994 Influenza Vaccines** *Tamar Lasky, PhD* *National Institute of Child Health & Human Development*
2:45 – 3:15 pm	**Safety of Influenza Vaccine in the Pediatric Population** *Eric K. France, MD, MSPH* *Preventive Medicine Kaiser Permanente Colorado*
3:15 – 3:30 pm	**Break**
3:30 – 4:00 pm	**Intranasal Vaccines** *Kathryn Edwards, MD, (presented via conference call)* *Vanderbilt University School of Medicine*
4:00 – 4:30 pm	**VSD Data Related to Influenza Vaccine and Incidence/Relapse of MS** *Frank DeStefano, MD* *Centers for Disease Control and Prevention*
4:30 – 4:45 pm	**Use of Medicare Data to Evaluate Adverse Events After Influenza Vaccine** *Dale Burwen, MD,* *Food and Drug Administration*
4:45 – 5:30 pm	**Discussion and Public Comment**
5:30 pm	**Adjourn**

Appendix C

Chronology of Important Events Regarding Vaccine Safety

Year	Vaccine Licensure	Legislation and/or Policy Statements	IOM Reports on Vaccine Safety
1955	Inactivated poliomyelitis vaccine (IPV) available		
1963	Oral poliomyelitis vaccine (OPV) available, replaces IPV		
	Measles vaccine available		
1967	Mumps vaccine available		
1969	Rubella vaccine available		
1971	Measles-Mumps-Rubella (MMR) vaccine available		
1977		Mumps vaccination recommended	*Evaluation of Poliomyelitis Vaccines*
1979	Current formulation of rubella vaccine available, replaces earlier versions		
1982	Plasma-derived hepatitis B vaccine available		

Year	Vaccine Licensure	Legislation and/or Policy Statements	IOM Reports on Vaccine Safety
1985	Hib vaccine licensed for children >15 months		
1986		Congress passes Public Law 99-660, the National Childhood Vaccine Injury Act (introduced in 1984) calls for: • est. of NVPO • est. of NVAC • est. of VICP • est. of ACCV IOM review of 1) pertussis and rubella, 2) routine child vaccines	
1988			*Evaluation of Poliomyelitis Vaccine Policy Options*
1990	2 Hib conjugate vaccines licensed for use beginning at 2 months		
1991	Acellular pertussis component licensed for the 4th and 5th doses of the 5-part DTP series in ACEL-IMUNE	Hepatitis B recommended by ACIP for addition to childhood immunization schedule ACIP recommends Hib be added to childhood immunization schedule	*Adverse Effects of Pertussis and Rubella Vaccines*
1992	Acellular pertussis component licensed for the 4th and 5th doses of the 5-part DTP series in Tripedia	Hepatitis B vaccine: Added universal vaccination for all infants, high-risk adolescents (e.g., IV drug users, persons with multiple sex partners)	
1993	Combined DTP and Hib vaccine (Tetramune) licensed		

Year	Vaccine Licensure	Legislation and/or Policy Statements	IOM Reports on Vaccine Safety
1994			*Adverse Events Associated with Childhood Vaccines: Evidence Bearing on Causality* *DPT and Chronic Nervous System Dysfunction: A New Analysis*
1995	Varicella virus vaccine available (Varivax)		
1996	DTaP vaccine licensed for first three doses given in infancy (Tripedia and ACEL-IMUNE were previously licensed for only the 4th and 5th doses).	ACIP recommends using IPV for the first 2 polio vaccinations, followed by OPV for remaining doses. Intended to be a transitional schedule for 3–5 years until an all-IPV series is available ACIP recommends children 12months – 12 years receive Varicella vaccine	*Options for Poliomyelitis Vaccinations in the United States: Workshop Summary*
1997	Additional DTaP vaccine (Infanrix) licensed for first 4 doses of 5-part series	ACIP recommends DTaP in place of DTP	*Vaccine Safety Forum: Summary of Two Workshops* *Risk Communication and Vaccination: Workshop Summary*
1998	Additional DTaP vaccine (Certiva) licensed for first 4 doses of 5-part series	ACIP updates MMR recommendation, encouraging use of the combined MMR vaccine	

Year	Vaccine Licensure	Legislation and/or Policy Statements	IOM Reports on Vaccine Safety
1999		ACIP updates varicella vaccine recommendation, requiring immunity for child care and school entry	
		ACIP recommends an all-IPV schedule begin January 2000 to prevent cases of vaccine-associated paralytic polio	
		AAP and PHS recommend removal of thimerosal from vaccines Also recommended postponement of hepatitis B vaccine from birth to 2–6 months for infants of hepatitis B surface antigen-negative mothers	
	Additional supply of thimerosal-free hepatitis B vaccine made available	*MMWR* notifies readers of the availability of a thimerosal-free hepatitis B vaccine, enabling the resumption of the birth dose	
2000	Pneumococcal vaccine for infants and young children licensed (Prevnar)	ACIP recommends pneumococcal vaccination for all children 2–23 months, and at-risk children 24–59 months (e.g., immunocompromised)	
2001		October: ACIP drafts statement expressing a preference for use of thimerosal-free DTaP, Hib, and Hep B vaccines by March 2002	*Immunization Safety Review: Measles-Mumps-Rubella Vaccine and Autism* *Immunization Safety Review: Thimerosal-Containing Vaccines and Neuro-developmental Disorders*

Year	Vaccine Licensure	Legislation and/or Policy Statements	IOM Reports on Vaccine Safety
2002			*Immunization Safety Review: Multiple Immunizations and Immune Dysfunction*
			Immunization Safety Review: Hepatitis B Vaccine and Demyelinating Neurological Disorders
			Immunization Safety Review: SV40 Contamination of Polio Vaccine and Cancer
2003	Live attenuated intranasal influenza vaccine approved for use in the United States in healthy individuals aged 5-49 years old (FluMist)	ACIP recommends that children 6 to 23 months of age be vaccinated annually against influenza beginning in the 2004-2005 influenza season	*Immunization Safety Review: Hepatitis B Vaccine and Demyelinating Neurological Disorders*
			Immunization Safety Review: SV40 Contamination of Polio Vaccine and Cancer
			Immunization Safety Review: Vaccinations and Sudden Unexpected Death in Infancy

Appendix D

Acronyms

AAN – American Academy of Neurologists
ACCV – Advisory Commission on Childhood Vaccines
ACIP – Advisory Committee on Immunization Practices
ADEM – acute disseminated encephalomyelitis
AIDP – acute inflammatory demyelinating polyradiculoneuropathy
AMAN – acute motor axonal neuropathy
AMSAN – acute motor sensory axonal neuropathy

CDC – Centers for Disease Control and Prevention
CI – confidence interval
CNS – central nervous system
CSF – cerebral spinal fluid

DNA – deoxyribonucleic acid

EAE – experimental autoimmune encephalomyelitis
EAN – experimental allergic neuritis
EN – experimental neuritis
EMG – electromyography
EPA – Environmental Protection Agency

FDA – Food and Drug Administration

GBS – Guillain-Barré syndrome

HA – hemagglutinin
HIV – human immunodeficiency virus
HMO – health maintenance organization

IAVG – Interagency Vaccine Group
ICD – 9 – International Classification of Diseases, Ninth Revision
IOM – Institute of Medicine
IM – intramuscular
IVIG – intravenous immunoglobulin
LOS – lipooligosaccharide
LPS – lipopolysaccharide

M – matrix proteins
MFS – Miller Fisher syndrome/ Fisher syndrome
MRI – magnetic resonance imaging
MS – multiple sclerosis

NA – neuraminidase
NCHS – National Center for Health Statistics
NP – nucleoprotein
NIH – National Institutes of Health
NVAC – National Vaccine Advisory Committee
NVPO – National Vaccine Program Office

OS – oligosaccharide

PNS – peripheral nervous system

RNA – ribonucleic acid
RRMS – relapsing-remitting multiple sclerosis

TMEV – Theiler's murine encephalomyelitis virus

USDA – United States Department of Agriculture

VAERS – Vaccine Adverse Event Reporting System
VICP – Vaccine Injury Compensation Program

WHO – World Health Organization